Practical Peripheral Arterial Thrombolysis

Practical Peripheral Arterial Thrombolysis

J. J. Earnshaw   MB, BS, DM, FRCS
Consultant Surgeon
Gloucestershire Royal Hospital
Gloucester, UK

R. H. S. Gregson   BSc, MB, BS, FRCR
Consultant Radiologist
University Hospital
Nottingham, UK

BUTTERWORTH
HEINEMANN

Butterworth-Heinemann Ltd
Linacre House, Jordan Hill, Oxford OX2 8DP

A member of the Reed Elsevier plc group

OXFORD   LONDON   BOSTON
MUNICH   NEW DELHI   SINGAPORE   SYDNEY
TOKYO   TORONTO   WELLINGTON

First published 1994

© Butterworth-Heinemann Ltd 1994

British Library Cataloguing in Publication Data

A catalogue record for this book is available from
the British Library

ISBN 0 7506 0757 2

Library of Congress Cataloging in Publication Data

A catalogue record for this book is available from
the Library of Congress

Filmset by P&R Typesetters Ltd, Salisbury, England
Printed in Great Britain at the University Press, Cambridge

Contents

Contributors

Jonathan D. Beard ChM FRCS
Consultant Surgeon, Royal Hallamshire Hospital, Sheffield

David C. Berridge DM FRCS
Senior Surgical Registrar, Freeman Hospital, Newcastle upon Tyne

Tim Buckenham FRACR
Consultant Radiologist, St George's Hospital, London

Kieran J. Dawson FRCS
Vascular Research Fellow, Royal Free Hospital, London

Jonothan J. Earnshaw DM FRCS
Consultant Surgeon, Gloucestershire Royal Hospital

Anthony E. B. Giddings MD FRCS
Consultant Surgeon, Royal Surrey County Hospital, Guildford

Roger H. S. Gregson BSc, MB, BS, FRCR
Consultant Radiologist, University Hospital, Nottingham

George Hamilton FRCS
Consultant Surgeon, Royal Free Hospital, London

Brian R. Hopkinson ChM FRCS
Consultant Surgeon, University Hospital, Nottingham

Robert J. Lonsdale FRCS
Surgical Registrar, University Hospital, Nottingham

Geoffrey S. Makin ChM FRCS
Consultant Surgeon, University Hospital, Nottingham

Ian S. Paterson MD FRCS
Consultant Surgeon, Good Hope Hospital, Birmingham

Clifford P. Shearman MS FRCS
Consultant Senior Lecturer in Surgery, Queen Elizabeth Hospital, Birmingham

Woodruff J. Walker FFR(SA) FRCR
Consultant Radiologist, Royal Surrey County Hospital, Guildford

Preface

Our aim was to produce a book that would appeal both to beginners at thrombolysis and also surgeons and radiologists with experience in thrombolytic techniques who wish to re-analyse their methods. It will become apparent to readers of this book that there is no single correct way to perform thrombolytic therapy but that all radiologists and surgeons have a slightly different approach. In this book, clinicians familiar with peripheral thrombolysis provide details of their methods together with an up-to-date assessment of techniques reported in the literature. Often contrasting techniques will be presented for a particular clinical situation and the reader will be left to adapt the method which is closest to his or her own style. Peripheral thrombolysis is still in its infancy and we all have much to learn from each other before we can be sure which techniques are optimal.

Jonothan J. Earnshaw
Roger H. S. Gregson

Introduction

We welcome the appearance of this monograph on a subject of increasing importance. Local thrombolysis is being regarded as a first line of therapy for many patients with acutely ischaemic limbs and it is now opportune to gather together the many threads of endeavour on the subject.

The joint authorship demonstrates the importance of teamwork in this area and close co-operation between surgeon and radiologist is essential for such techniques to succeed. We are equal colleagues with our radiologists in managing these patients.

The evolution of new thrombolytic agents and methods of delivery is proceeding rapidly. The possible combination with adjuvant anti-platelet agents is a subject still to be resolved.

What is the role of surgery? Many patients require surgery or angioplasty in addition, but we will have to await the outcome of properly controlled trials containing large numbers of patients before we know which is superior. In any case, have we yet achieved the ideal thrombolytic regime? We hope this publication will set the scene.

G. S. Makin
B. R. Hopkinson

Chapter 1

Introduction to fibrinolysis

J. J. Earnshaw

Fibrinolysis

Historical aspects of fibrinolysis

The earliest observations on the physiology of the fibrinolytic system date back to 1769 when Morgagni observed whilst performing the post-mortem of a young man who had been stabbed in the heart, that his blood was not clotted, but fluid. He misinterpreted that this was caused by the large quantity of alcohol the man had consumed prior to his death[1]. Similarly, John Hunter (1794) noted that the blood of stags chased to their death was incoagulable. He recognized that menstrual blood did not coagulate and believed that these findings were due to 'some property inherent in the blood itself'. Others including Virchow (1871) noted that post-mortem blood was fluid and in 1893 Dastre observed that normal blood clots eventually redissolved and coined the term of 'fibrinolysis' for this occurrence[2]. It was not until 1933 that Tillett and Garner at the Rockefeller Institute stimulated renewed interest in fibrinolysis when they discovered that cell filtrates from certain haemolytic streptococci contained a substance which dissolved fibrin[3]. They isolated this substance and demonstrated in a series of experiments that fibrin clots were only susceptible to lysis by this factor in the presence of a plasma factor they called the lytic agent. This proved subsequently to be plasminogen. Christenson (1945) continued these experiments and termed the substance produced by streptococci – streptokinase[4]. Now there was an agent with which to perform studies, and in a series of experiments the plasma fibrinolytic system was thoroughly evaluated over the next few years. MacFarlane and Pilling (1947) isolated a second plasminogen activator from human urine which they termed urokinase[5]. Later still, Mullertz (1953) demonstrated that a third plasminogen activator was released from human veins after exogenous stimuli[6]. He termed this agent vascular plasminogen activator, though it has subsequently become known as tissue plasminogen activator (t-PA).

The importance of plasma fibrinolytic activity

It has been demonstrated that small quantities of fibrin are produced as a by-product of wear and tear on vascular endothelium. The plasma fibrinolytic system is the mechanism by which this is removed. Astrup (1958) described the 'haemostatic balance' by which vascular patency was maintained[7]. Any alteration in this haemostatic balance caused either by reduced plasma fibrinolytic activity or an increased tendency to coagulation might cause pathological thrombosis. Plasma fibrinolytic activity has been extensively investigated and has been shown to have a diurnal variation. Fibrinolytic activity is increased by exercise, alcohol and some drugs including vasopressin and oral hypoglycaemic agents, but is depressed by smoking and in patients with diabetes mellitus or hypertriglyceridaemia[8].

It has been shown that the plasma fibrinolytic system is defective in many common thrombotic diseases. Reduced fibrinolytic activity may have a role in spontaneous deep vein thrombosis (DVT), though a significant effect has been more clearly demonstrated in patients with recurrent DVT[9]. Abnormal pre-operative plasma fibrinolytic activity can be used to predict the likelihood of post-operative DVT[10]. Fibrinolytic activity has also been shown to be defective in patients with peripheral arterial disease[11] and acute myocardial infarction[12]. However, it is not clear whether the reduced plasma fibrinolytic activity in these patients is a cause or an effect of the disease.

Components of the fibrinolytic system (Figure 1.1)

PLASMINOGEN/PLASMIN

Plasminogen is a glycoprotein synthesized in the liver. Its structure contains five triple loop regions called kringles which contain the lysine binding sites that interact with fibrin and anti-plasmins. Plasminogen activators react with plasminogen to form active plasmin which then binds strongly to any available fibrin. Plasmin is a non-specific proteolytic enzyme which can digest many proteins including fibrin and fibrinogen. The presence of plasma inhibitors mops up any circulating plasmin and confers a relative specificity for fibrin, whilst sparing fibrinogen. Thus plasmin has a very short half-life in the circulation before it is inactivated and only a very small amount can be measured in plasma.

PLASMINOGEN ACTIVATORS

Endogenous activators occur naturally in blood and other body tissues and fluids. These include urokinase, pro-urokinase and t-PA. Exogenous activators such as streptokinase are produced artificially and given for therapeutic effect.

Tissue plasminogen activator
Tissue plasminogen activator is produced by vascular endothelial cells of both arteries and veins and is responsible for plasma fibrinolytic activity. It is also produced by many cells in other body tissues and may have important roles in prevention of spread of infection and tumour growth. t-PA has a short half-life in plasma of 2–5 minutes, and is metabolized rapidly by the liver. Activity of plasma t-PA is reduced by a specific inhibitor – plasminogen activator inhibitor (PAI). There is very little free circulating t-PA due to the extraordinarily high affinity of PAI. Most measurable plasma t-PA exists in complex with PAI and is inactive. Free circulating t-PA has a high affinity for plasminogen in the presence of fibrin. This affinity is mediated through the two kringles in its structure[13].

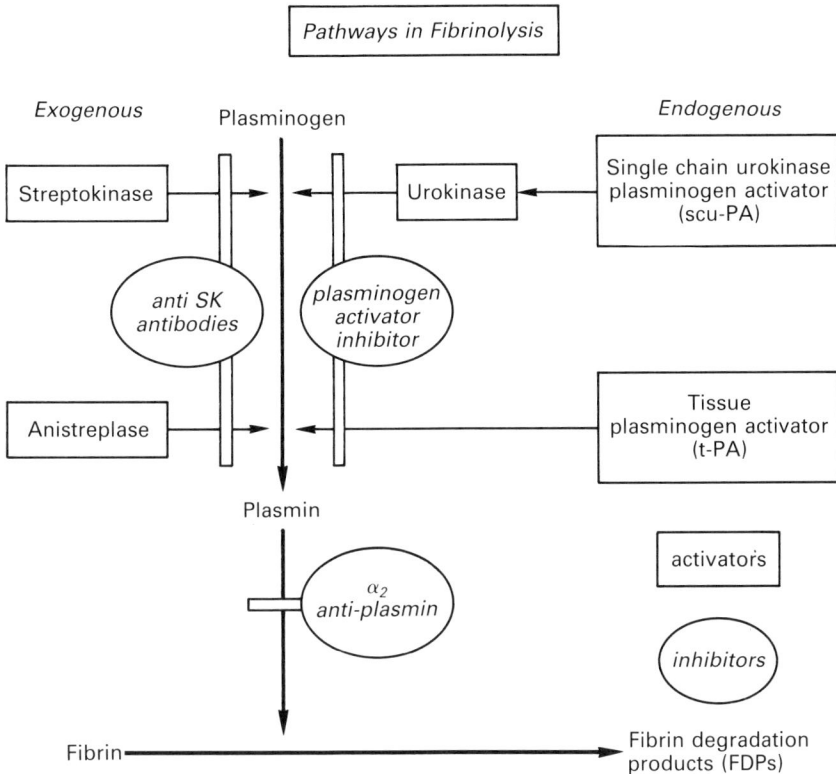

Figure 1.1 Pathways in fibrinolysis

Urokinase
Urokinase was initially discovered in the urine by MacFarlane and Pilling (in 1947)[5], but is also present in many other cells. It can be demonstrated immunologically in plasma and probably also plays a part in the maintenance of plasma fibrinolytic activity, although its exact importance is uncertain. A pre-activator, pro-urokinase, has recently been discovered and is inactive in plasma, but in the presence of fibrin is converted to urokinase. It is presently termed single chain urokinase plasminogen activator (scu-PA). Urokinase, unlike streptokinase, is a direct activator of plasminogen and does not require co-factors. It is non-antigenic[14].

Streptokinase
Streptokinase is an exogenous plasminogen activator produced as a by-product of certain beta haemolytic streptococci. This has the disadvantage of rendering it antigenic in humans. Most individuals have antibodies in the plasma due to previous infection with streptococci. These antibodies bind rapidly to streptokinase rendering it inactive. The antibodies can be overcome by giving a loading dose of streptokinase, but maintenance infusion results in an increasing antibody response which reduces the effectiveness of long-term treatment. The mechanism of action of streptokinase is indirect.

Plasminogen is required as a co-activator to form an activator complex which converts plasminogen to plasmin. It was discovered that the co-activator is plasminogen itself because the maximum fibrinolytic activity occurs when streptokinase and plasminogen are present in equimolar concentrations.

INHIBITORS OF FIBRINOLYSIS

The plasma fibrinolytic system has many inhibitors but the two most physiologically important are alpha-2-antiplasmin and the plasminogen activator inhibitors.

Alpha-2-antiplasmin
Alpha-2-antiplasmin is the most important inhibitor of plasmin. Although it has a low concentration in normal plasma it has a very strong affinity for plasmin, rendering the half-life of circulating plasmin very short and preventing its general systemic effects. Other plasmin inhibitors such as alpha-2-macroglobulin, alpha-1-antitrypsin, C1-esterase inhibitor and anti-thrombin III have lesser roles to play.

Plasminogen activator inhibitor (PAI)
This group of compounds has only recently been discovered and is still under evaluation. PAIs interact specifically with plasminogen activators to block activity. They are secreted from the liver and vascular endothelium and four subspecies are presently under investigation. PAI-1 is the best understood and is present in small concentrations in plasma where it reacts very quickly to neutralize t-PA or urokinase. PAI-2 is predominantly intracellular and inhibits plasminogen activation during pregnancy. Less still is known about PAI-3 and PAI-4. The majority of circulating t-PA exists as a complex with PAI which renders it inactive. In the presence of fibrin, t-PA is protected from PAI and is thus available to activate plasminogen[15]. Alterations in PAI levels may be the most important cause for variations in plasma fibrinolytic activity both in health and disease. Elevated PAI levels have been shown to be the main cause of defective plasma fibrinolytic activity in thrombotic disease, such as DVT and myocardial infarction[16], and to cause the well-known effect of 'fibrinolytic shutdown' after surgery. It is not known, however, whether elevated PAI levels are a cause or an effect of thrombotic disease. PAI behaves like an acute phase reaction protein in response to infection or trauma.

Response to intravascular thrombosis

Intravascular coagulation results in fibrin production. Specific binding sites on fibrin attract circulating plasminogen activators, and probably also those released locally in response to vessel injury. Plasminogen activators – t-PA and also probably urokinase – bind specifically to fibrin. The reaction of binding uncovers other binding sites on the activator molecule which react with plasminogen bound within the thrombus to convert it locally to plasmin, resulting in degradation of the fibrin. Any free circulating t-PA is mopped up by PAI and any free plasmin is inactivated by alpha-2-antiplasmin. Therefore this fibrinolytic reaction is localized at the site of the thrombus and the importance of plasminogen trapped within the thrombus is also evident.

The action of the plasma fibrinolytic system is apparent in the normal recanalization of forearm veins which thrombose after venepuncture or varicose veins which recanalize after thrombophlebitis. Recanalization often occurs after DVT, although the damage produced in the deep venous valves results in deep venous insufficiency. The process of fibrinolysis after major thrombosis is slow. It can be demonstrated in the arterial circulation where small emboli may lyse spontaneously, but natural fibrinolysis is often too late to prevent death after myocardial infarction or limb loss following acute arterial occlusion.

Systemic fibrinolysis

Systemic fibrinolysis never occurs naturally but is the response to administration of thrombolytic agents or abnormal production of plasminogen activators. The effect of thrombolytic agents given either intravenously or intra-arterially is similar. The response depends on the concentration of agent given and on the level of plasma inhibition. At the lowest concentration, plasminogen is converted to plasmin which will degrade any fibrinogen or fibrin in the area of infusion. Any circulating plasmin will be inactivated by alpha-2-antiplasmin. Increasing levels of fibrinolytic agent will cause all plasminogen to be converted to plasmin, overwhelming the normal inhibition mechanism and causing systemic plasminaemia. At this concentration circulating fibrinogen is degraded. Initially this does not appear to matter and indeed may enhance critical ischaemia by improving blood viscosity. However, when plasma fibrinogen levels fall below 1 g/dl spontaneous bleeding may occur and the risk of haemorrhagic complications increases. Both fibrin and fibrinogen breakdown result in the appearance of fibrin(ogen) degradation products (FDP). FDPs are themselves anticoagulant and further potentiate the risk of bleeding. When a systemic fibrinolytic state exists, circulating plasminogen is depleted and any further thrombosis (such as pericatheter thrombosis or rethrombosis during thrombolysis) will not contain plasminogen which reduces its susceptibility to further lysis.

The extent of systemic fibrinolysis during thrombolytic therapy is determined by the concentration and specificity of the agent. Streptokinase is not fibrin specific, but endogenous agents such as t-PA and urokinase have specific binding sites for fibrin. When plasminogen is activated by t-PA the resulting complex binds locally to thrombus and acts specifically at that site. This reduces the systemic effects, although a degree of systemic activity is always recordable. Fibrinogen degradation is delayed and reduced by the clinical use of fibrin-specific thrombolytic agents. However, there appears to be a cumulative effect and prolonged infusion of fibrin-specific thrombolytic agents eventually causes systemic activation.

It was hoped that fibrin-specific agents would make thrombolytic treatment safer and more effective than using streptokinase. Fibrin specificity should reduce systemic activation over a wider range of infusion concentrations. However, thrombolytic drugs cannot differentiate between useful fibrin clots sealing vessels and harmful thrombus occluding important vessels. The more specific the thrombolytic agent, the higher the risk of a useful fibrin plug being lysed, potentially increasing the risk of complications such as stroke or retroperitoneal haemorrhage. Clinical trials are required to establish the risk and complications of each thrombolytic agent.

Treatment of systemic fibrinolysis

Rarely, patients may have a bleeding disorder due to congenitally high t-PA levels or malignant tumours which secrete plasminogen activators. Other unusual causes of systemic fibrinolytic activation include disseminated intravascular coagulation and venom from some snake bites. The most common cause of bleeding due to excess fibrinolytic activity is the clinical application of thrombolytic agents. Patients with systemic fibrinolysis may have spontaneous haemorrhage and require intensive treatment with blood transfusion and coagulation factors. Transfusion of clotting factors in fresh frozen plasma may help the generalized coagulation disorder but the most important agent to consider is cryoprecipitate which replenishes fibrinogen levels, the principal cause of haemorrhage. Drugs which inhibit the fibrinolytic system may be used, including tranexamic acid (Cyklokapron, Kabi Pharmaceuticals) or aprotinin (Trasylol, Bayer). Tranexamic acid forms a reversible complex with plasminogen which prevents its activation, whereas aprotinin forms a reversible complex with plasmin itself.

In the event of uncontrolled bleeding from systemic fibrinolysis, the best advice is to administer both fresh frozen plasma together with cryoprecipitate and one of the above anti-fibrinolytic drugs. Regular monitoring of coagulation is required to avoid overcorrection.

Early clinical use of thrombolytic therapy

The first studies of thrombolytic therapy in thrombotic diseases used non-specific proteolytic enzymes such as trypsin and plasmin[17]. There was little effect and a high complication rate when either of these treatments was given intravenously. It became apparent that successful thrombolysis required activation of fibrin-bound plasminogen. Clinical therapy was therefore better with a plasminogen activator than with plasmin itself. The discovery of streptokinase by Tillett and Garner in 1933[3] gave rise to a specific plasminogen activator for clinical use. Streptokinase was initially very impure and it was not until 20 years after its discovery that it was first suitable for intravenous administration in clinical studies. Following extensive investigation of thrombosis in animal models, streptokinase was first tested in patients with loculated haemothorax following pneumonectomy, enabling the liquefield blood to be drained[18]. In 1959 Johnson and McCarty demonstrated lysis of artificially induced peripheral thrombosis in forearm veins of humans using streptokinase[19]. It was then that the potential for thrombolytic therapy as a treatment of thrombotic disease became apparent. Myocardial infarction, deep venous thrombosis, pulmonary embolism and acute peripheral arterial ischaemia are among the commonest causes of human suffering and the potential for thrombolytic therapy is immense.

Acute leg ischaemia

Historical aspects of acute leg ischaemia

Atherosclerotic limb ischaemia was rare before the twentieth century. In one of a series of surgical lectures published in *The Lancet* in 1823, Sir Astley Cooper stated that gangrene was usually due to infection or trauma and occasionally an aneurysm. He stated that less frequently gangrene occurred 'in old persons . . . from ossification of the arteries . . . combined with a debilitated action of the heart. Earthy matter (atheroma) sometimes is deposited in great quantities in the large vessels'[20]. The only available treatment for painful gangrene was amputation which carried a high mortality and was usually avoided at all costs. Most amputations up until the twentieth century were for trauma. Knowledge about acute limb ischaemia derived from the treatment of vascular trauma and also from primary arterial ligation, a technique which was developed for the treatment of peripheral aneurysms. John Hunter was among the first to treat limb aneurysms with simple arterial ligation. His well-recorded treatment of a popliteal aneurysm in a coachman in 1785 is the famous example[21]. It was recognized by Kirkes in 1852 that acute ischaemia was frequently caused by embolic material[22]. He noted 'fibrinous concretions on the valves of the interior of the heart admit of being readily detached during life, and mingling with the circulating blood . . . if detached and transmitted in large masses they may suddenly block up the large artery, and so cut off the supply of blood to an important part'. The term embolus was coined by Virchow (1854) and the association between endocarditis and embolism was recorded[23].

Surgery for acute leg ischaemia

Direct arterial surgery was not practised until the early twentieth century, although Hallowell (1761) is credited with the first arterial suture when he repaired a lacerated brachial artery with a pin and ligature[24]. In 1894 Severeanu of Bucharest recommended probing the popliteal artery with an oiled catheter during an amputation to remove any residual thrombus in the hope of encouraging the skin flaps to heal[25]. The first direct embolectomy was performed by Ssabanajeff (1895) though it was not successful[26]. Others also reported failed attempts. In 1911 two surgeons, Georges Labey in Paris[27] and Einar Key in Stockholm[28], performed successful operations for femoral emboli of less than 6 hours' duration. The technique was slow to be adopted and there were still only 129 cases in the English-speaking literature by 1933[29]. Many techniques were used over the next 30 years to try and improve surgical embolectomy including retrograde massage of the limb using an Esmarch type tourniquet, a distal arteriotomy with prolonged saline flushing, and the use of a corkscrew wire or an olive head vein stripper. Results using these techniques were, at best, modest. Other improvements which were incorporated into the management of acute limb ischaemia included the use of anticoagulants. Heparin was introduced in the 1930s[30] and warfarin in the 1940s[31] as means of preventing rethrombosis after embolectomy.

The greatest surgical advance was the development of the balloon embolectomy catheter by Thomas Fogarty in 1963[32]. This had the advantage that, in expert hands, little intimal damage was caused and yet secondary thrombus could be removed from a site distant to an arteriotomy. Immediate improvements in the outcome from acute leg ischaemia were reported with the use of this technique[33]. In the 1950s and 1960s came the development of arterial reconstructive techniques, both with autogenous vein and synthetic grafts. These techniques became alternatives for patients in whom thrombus could not be removed by an embolectomy catheter, and those with associated arterial occlusive disease.

Clinical aspects of acute arterial occlusion

Sudden total occlusion of a normal artery by, for example, a cardiac embolus results in an acute white leg with the classic symptoms and signs of:

—pain
—pulselessness
—paraesthesia
—pallor
—paralysis
—perishing with cold

Initially the leg is marble white and the veins empty and guttered. Over the next 12 hours, vasodilatation occurs and the veins refill and pool blood resulting in a blue mottled appearance. This is a grim sign which implies impending tissue death and necrosis. If the ischaemia is unrelieved, capillary rupture occurs resulting in fixed blue staining of the skin. Other signs of irreversible ischaemia include muscle turgor and tenderness (Figure 1.2).

Revascularization of ischaemic tissue may be dangerous in the latter stages of the above process. Initially toxic metabolites may be introduced into the general circulation which result in systemic hyperkalaemia and acidosis thus increasing susceptibility to cardiac arrhythmias. Revascularization of necrotic muscle can introduce myoglobin into the circulation causing myoglobinuria and renal failure[34]. Later other effects of revascularization become apparent including activation of neutrophils and production of oxygen free radicals, causing further local and systemic damage. These effects are discussed in Chapter 2.

Often the arterial occlusion is not so catastrophic, particularly if the occlusion is not total or sudden so that a collateral circulation has had time to develop. This is particularly the case in arterial thrombosis where thrombus often supervenes on a pre-existing arterial stenosis (Figure 1.3) In this case the clinical signs may be more subtle, indeed the event may even be asymptomatic. Pain is often a feature and there may be a degree of sensory loss without total paralysis. This situation is termed acute-on-chronic ischaemia. Clinical examination will reveal loss of peripheral pulses and ankle

0–6 hours	6–12 hours	over 12 hours
Painful, marble white foot Neurosensory deficit	Mottled appearance due to capillary pooling Blanches on digital pressure	Fixed staining: mottled areas coalesce and no longer blanch to pressure Anterior compartment red and tender
Reversible	Partly reversible	Irreversible

(a)

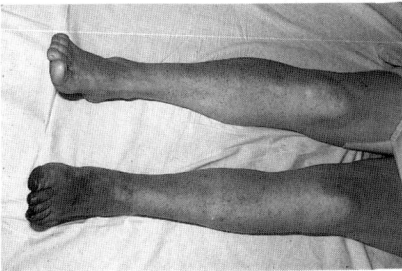 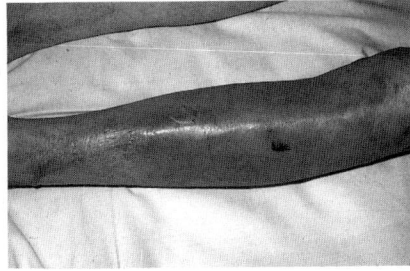

(b)   (c)

Figure 1.2 (a) Clinical events in acute leg ischaemia. (b) Mottled fixed staining of an ischaemic leg implies irreversible ischaemia. (c) Discoloured anterior compartment implies muscle necrosis

Doppler pressure measurements may be helpful in diagnosis. In these cases time is not so critical in restoring the circulation before muscle necrosis occurs. This is in contrast with acute total ischaemia where irreversible muscle necrosis may occur in as little as 6 hours.

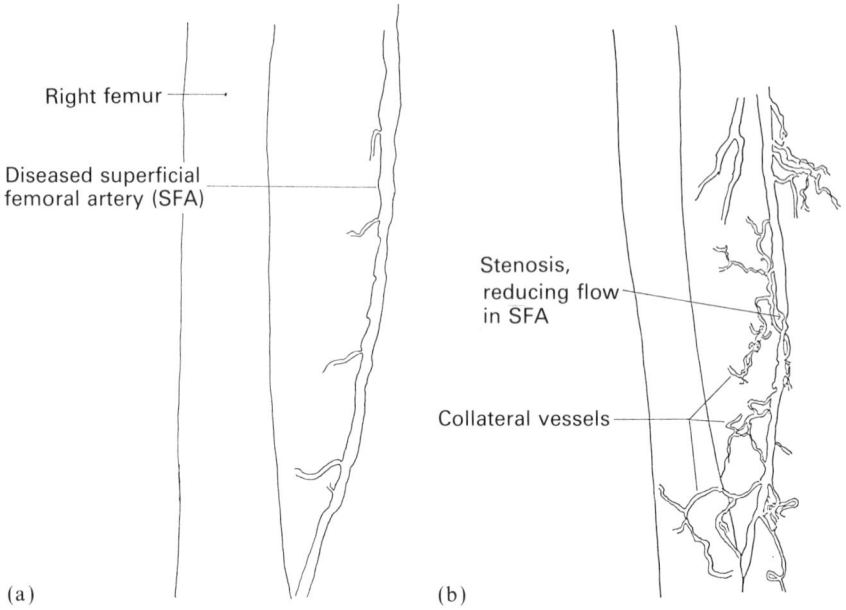

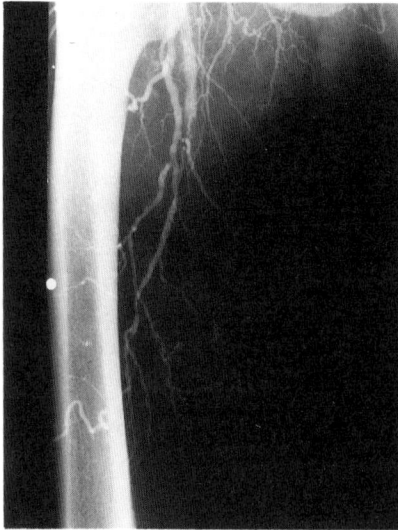

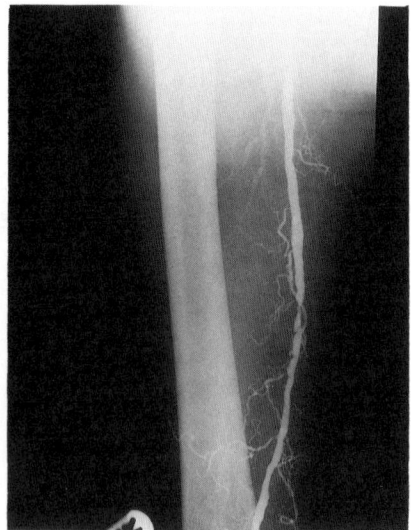

(a)

Right femur

Diseased superficial
femoral artery (SFA)

(b)

Stenosis,
reducing flow
in SFA

Collateral vessels

(d)

(e)

Surgical management of acute leg ischaemia

It is widely reported that there are differences in outcome when patients with
acute thrombosis or embolism are compared. Surgery for acute thrombosis
results in a higher amputation rate because of thrombus involving distal
vessels. Embolectomy is associated with a higher mortality due to existing

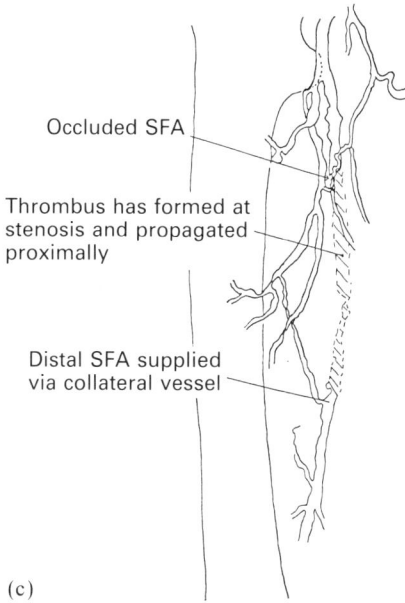

Occluded SFA

Thrombus has formed at
stenosis and propagated
proximally

Distal SFA supplied
via collateral vessel

(c)

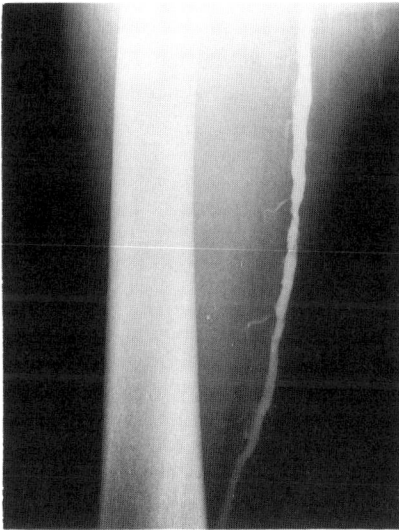

(f)

Figure 1.3 Pathophysiology of acute
thrombosis: uncovered by thrombolysis.
(a) Early generalized superficial femoral artery
artherosclerosis with developing collaterals.
(b) Stenosis develops at mid-point of
superficial femoral artery with restricted
femoral flow increasing collaterals.
(c) Platelets and fibrin collect on stenosis and
result in occlusion. Collateral vessels restore
flow to distal superficial femoral artery.
(d) Acute superficial femoral artery
thrombosis. (e) Superficial femoral artery,
recanalized by low-dose streptokinase
uncovering mid-point stenosis. (f) Good
flow after successful angioplasty

cardiac disease which often produced the embolus[35,36]. For this reason
surgeons have attempted to make a preoperative diagnosis. An embolus is
usually associated with a clinically obvious source such as atrial fibrillation,
cardiac valve disease or myocardial infarction. There is rarely pre-existing
peripheral arterial disease. Acute thrombosis is often associated with a prior

history of intermittent claudication or other atherosclerotic disease. In the presence of an embolus, distal vessels are usually normal and embolectomy, particularly if performed promptly under local anaesthesia, often gives a good result. Acute thrombosis occurs when thrombus supervenes on a pre-existing stenosed segment of artery. Embolectomy in this situation often adds further intimal damage and results in amputation[37]. Embolectomy reserved for strict criteria – a duration less than 24 hours, an obvious source and no prior claudication – dramatically reduces the number performed but improves outcome considerably[38]. Patients with acute thromboses should have an urgent vascular assessment, which is best performed by trained vascular surgeons, followed by an angiogram[39]. Prompt surgery in these cases can result in a good outcome but expert radiological and surgical facilities are beneficial. It is no longer acceptable simply to perform an embolectomy on all cases of acute leg ischaemia in the hope that some are emboli and will do well. A detailed assessment in a specialized unit yields better results[40].

Limitations of an aggressive surgical policy

Urgent surgery has been the traditional approach to the management of acute leg ischaemia. New techniques have altered this and thrombolysis and other non-surgical methods play a variable role in present management depending on the experience and enthusiasm of each individual clinician. Some authors continue to adopt an all-surgery policy and this can be evaluated in the light of current changes in patient profile.

In a consecutive 5-year series from Birmingham, 62 patients with severe acute ischaemia were reviewed. Embolectomy alone was successful in fewer than one-third; two-thirds required additional vascular reconstructive surgery. The result was a limb salvage rate of 62% and mortality of 19% after reconstruction and 33% after embolectomy alone[41]. A similar series from Portland, Oregon reported 72 patients treated over the same period: 20% had limbs beyond salvage and over half these patients died. In the remainder limb salvage was achieved in 87%, over 50% by inflow procedures alone. Interestingly, late mortality was 45% after 17 months in his series[42].

In both these reports, the majority of patients had acute thrombosis and were not suitable for embolectomy alone. This surgical approach results in long and often complex operations with high morbidity and mortality. Skilled vascular surgeons are needed and the cost of the surgery is high. Some of these patients may have avoided the physiological stresses of surgery if treated with thrombolysis. Formal randomized trials comparing surgery and thrombolysis have not yet been performed.

Surgery is better established for patients thought to have emboli. In the largest series published, including Fogarty's own results, over 700 embolectomies were performed[43]. In this selected group only 14% required additional vascular reconstruction with a limb salvage rate of 95% in survivors. The mortality rate was 12%. If an arterial stenosis is detected by intra-operative angiography after thromboembolectomy, on-table angioplasty can be performed. In a small series of 18 patients reported recently by Fogarty this was successful in 15, though three required additional inflow procedures[44]. Increasingly sophisticated technology and other endovascular techniques, such as angioscopic embolectomy[45], may expand the options available to surgeons treating patients with acute limb ischaemia.

A formal surgical approach to acute leg ischaemia is a reasonable option although there are problems (outlined above). There are serious limitations which suggest that the optimal approach is a selective one with a role for thrombolysis. The main reason that surgical enthusiasts dismiss thrombolysis is the time taken for it to be effective. Accelerated methods of thrombolysis can expand the indications to include patients with severe ischaemia and may encourage the surgical enthusiasts to alter their approach.

The high mortality resulting from urgent surgery for acute limb ischaemia (25% in a large collected series) was noted by Blaisdell who adopted an alternative, entirely conservative approach. He proposed anticoagulation with heparin as primary treatment for all patients whose limbs were not immediately threatened[46]. After 48 hours, patients with non-viable limbs had an amputation and the remainder had angiography with a view to planned vascular reconstruction. This method avoided high risk revascularization of limbs which had been ischaemic for 10–15 hours and 'traded limbs for lives'. In the series of 54 cases 28% required amputation although the mortality rate of 7% was very low. This again represents an extreme view which has been modified by others to be less drastic and provide good clinical results[47].

Thrombolysis for acute leg ischaemia

Following the purification of streptokinase for clinical use and initial studies in venous thrombosis and myocardial infarction, a few patients were treated with intra-arterial streptokinase (Figure 1.4). Cotton from King's College Hospital reported the first case in *The Lancet*[48]. A patient who had rethrombosis following femoral embolectomy received a total of 106 000 u streptokinase via an arterial catheter over 5 hours with a successful outcome. McNicol from Glasgow reported two similar cases, one in the brachial artery, for which larger doses were given, 12 500 u/h and 20 000 u/h, with success. McNicol also reported the use of streptokinase for subclavian vein thrombosis[49]. Clark also reported two cases and was the first to observe that age of occlusion and severity of ischaemia were important determinants of outcome[50]. In a Hunterian Lecture in 1964 Tsapogas reported eight cases and suggested that in future high dose infusions given through catheters with multiple side holes would be the best method[51].

Bleeding complications were frequent in early reports because the infusion catheters were bulky and inflexible. Imaging facilities and techniques were crude, vascular radiology was still in its infancy. Although a handful of successful cases were reported, the technique was not readily adopted. During the late 1960s intravenous streptokinase was evaluated for acute leg ischaemia and dosage schedules were refined. Several reports were published showing lysis rates of about 30% (see Chapter 3).

The revolution occurred with the development of the embolectomy catheter by Thomas Fogarty. This enabled distant thrombus to be retrieved through a groin incision and was widely adopted. The difficulties of embolectomy alluded to in the previous section encouraged further research into alternatives for acute leg ischaemia.

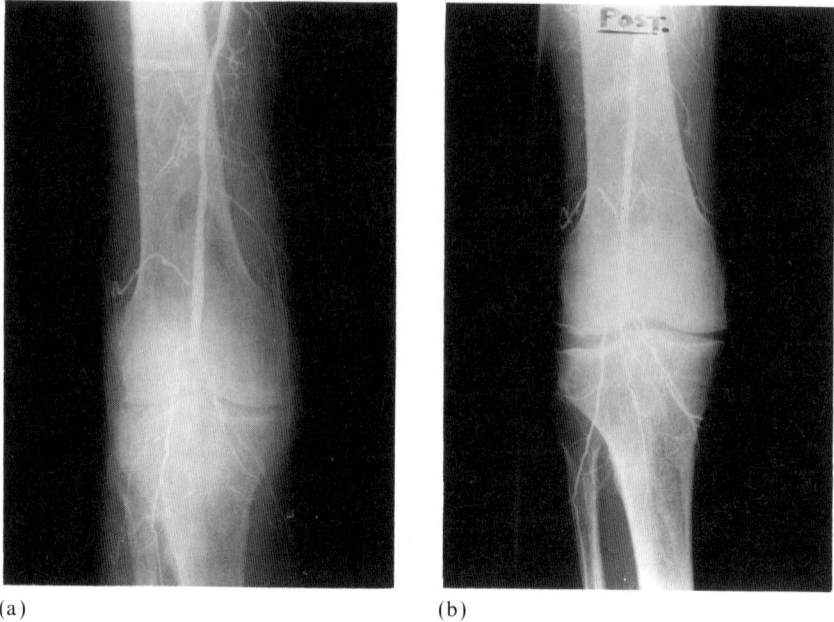

(a)   (b)

Figure 1.4 Early use of streptokinase (1962). (By kind permission of Professor N. Browse, PRCS.) (a) Acute popliteal artery embolism treated with intravenous streptokinase. (b) Some improvement after 72 hours. Patient left hospital with intact limb but subsequently required amputation

The first report of the use of low dose streptokinase came from Hirsch in 1969. In order to avoid systemic fibrinolysis in a patient with thrombocytopenia, a dose of 10 000 u/h was used in a patient with femoral artery thrombosis[52]. Chesterman reported a single case of distal arterial occlusion treated with streptokinase at 5000 u/h in 1971[53]. Charles Dotter from the University of Oregon is generally credited with the first major evaluation of local low dose streptokinase therapy for the treatment of acute leg ischaemia and standardized the dose at 5000 u/h[54]. However, it was not until 1982 when Hess from Munich published a report of 132 cases in the *New England Journal of Medicine* with lysis rates far superior to intravenous streptokinase that widespread interest in the method developed[55]. Subsequently, many surgeons and radiologists have recognized the potential of thrombolysis and the literature is full of reports of low dose intra-arterial streptokinase in the management of acute limb ischaemia. The importance of case selection has become evident and the severity of ischaemia at presentation is known to be the main limiting factor. It is interesting that most of the reports are uncontrolled and few randomized evaluations exist, yet intra-arterial thrombolysis has become firmly established as an alternative to surgery in the management of acute limb ischaemia[56].

With the burgeoning popularity of the technique, so have its limitations been exposed. The main problem is the length of time taken for effective thrombolysis, often 24–48 hours. In the last few years interest has returned to increasing the dose of thrombolytic agent to try and accelerate lysis. Several authors have reported methods which can reduce treatment to as few as 4 hours. Smaller arterial catheters, and improving technology, together with safer thrombolytic agents and monitoring, have combined to make accelerated thrombolysis a viable alternative to surgery. This dramatically increases the indications to include almost all cases of acute leg ischaemia. The principal treatment of acute limb ischaemia may now become medical rather than surgical.

Peripheral thrombolysis is a rapidly changing subject and the remainder of this book will review present knowledge and look towards the future and optimal management of patients with acute leg ischaemia.

References

1. Morgagni JB. *The Seats and Causes of Diseases*. London 1769; Vol. 3; Book 4; Letter 53: 185
2. Dastre A. Fibrinolyse dans la sang. *Arch Physiol Norm Pathol Paris* 1893; **5**: 661–3
3. Tillett WS and Garner RL. The fibrinolytic activity of haemolytic streptococci. *J Exp Med* 1933; **58**: 485–502
4. Christenson LR and MacLeod CM. Proteolytic enzymes of serum; characterization, activation and reaction with inhibitors. *J Gen Physiol* 1945; **28**: 559–83
5. MacFarlane RG and Pilling J. Fibrinolytic activity of normal urine. *Nature* 1947; **4049**: 779
6. Mullertz S. Plasminogen activator in spontaneously active human blood. *Proc Soc Exp Biol Med* 1953; **82**: 291–5
7. Astrup T. The haemostatic balance. *Thromb Diath Haemorrh* 1958; **2**: 347–57
8. Fearnley GR. Natural fibrinolysis. In: *Fibrinolysis*. Edward Arnold, London, 1965
9. Korninger C, Lechner K, Niessner H, Gossinger H and Kundi M. Impaired fibrinolytic capacity predisposes for recurrence of venous thrombosis. *Thromb Haemost* 1984; **52**: 127–30
10. Sue-Ling H. Johnston D, McMahon MJ, Philips PR and Davies JA. Pre-operative identification of patients at high risk of deep venous thrombosis after elective major abdominal surgery. *Lancet* 1986; **i**: 1173–6
11. Earnshaw JJ, Westby JC, Hopkinson BR and Makin GS. Resting plasma fibrinolytic activity and fibrinolytic potential in peripheral vascular disease. *J Cardiovasc Surg* 1988; **29**: 300–5
12. Estelles A, Tormo G, Aznar J, Espana F and Tormo V. Reduced fibrinolytic activity in coronary heart disease in basal conditions and after exercise. *Thromb Res* 1985; **40**: 373–83
13. Collen D and Lijnen HR. Basic clinical aspects of fibrinolysis and thrombolysis. *Blood* 1991; **78**: 3114–24
14. Lijnen HR, Van Hoef B, De Cock F and Collen D. The mechanism of action of plasminogen activation and fibrin dissolution by urokinase-type plasminogen activator in a plasma milieu in vitro. *Blood* 1989; **73**: 1864
15. Kruithof EKO. Plasminogen activator inhibitors – a review. *Enzyme* 1988; **40**: 113–21
16. Paramo JA, Colucci M, Collen D and Van de Werf F. Plasminogen activator inhibitor in the blood of patients with coronary heart disease. *Br Med J* 1985; **291**: 573–4
17. Laufman H and Roach HD. Intravenous trypsin in the treatment of thrombotic phenomena. *Arch Surg* 1953; **66**: 552–61
18. Tillett WS and Sherry S. The effect in patients of streptococcal fibrinolysin (streptokinase) and streptococcal desoxyribonuclease on fibrinous, purulent and sanguinous pleural exudations. *J Clin Invest* 1949; **28**: 173
19. Johnson AJ and McCarty WR. The lysis of artificially induced intravascular clots in mankind by intravenous infusions of streptokinase. *J Clin Invest* 1959; **38**: 1627–43
20. Cooper A. Surgical lectures. 15: Gangrene. *Lancet* 1823; **1; 9**: 289–300 and **10**: 321–8
21. Home E. An account of Mr Hunter's method of performing the operation for popliteal aneurysm. *London Med J* 1786; **7**: 391–406
22. Kirkes WS. On some of the principal effects resulting from the detachment of fibrinous deposits from the interior of the heart and their mixture with the circulating blood. *Med-Chi Trans* 1852

23. Virchow R. *Beitraege zur speziellen Pathologie und Therapie*, 1854
24. Hallowell. Cited by Lambert in: Erichsen JE (ed) *Observations on Aneurysm*. Sydenham Society, London, 1844: 265
25. Severeanu. Du catheterisme des arteres. *Prog Med* 1894: 89–90
26. Ssabanajeff. On the question of blood vessel suture. *Russk Khir Arkh* 1895: **11**: 625–39
27. Mosny M and Dumont NJ. Embolie femorale au cours d'un retrecissment mitral pour arteriotomie: guerison. *Bull Acad Natl Med* 1911; **56**: 358–61
28. Key E. Embolectomy in the treatment of circulatory disturbances in the extremities. *Surg Gynaecol Obstet* 1923; **36**: 309
29. Danzis M. Arterial embolectomy. *Ann Surg* 1933; **98**: 249–72, 422–37
30. Murray GDW, Jaques LB, Perrett TS and Best CH. Heparin and vascular occlusion. *Can Med Assoc J* 1936; **35**: 621–2
31. Butt HR, Allen EV and Bollman JL. Preparation from spoiled sweet clover which prolongs coagulation and prothrombin time of blood; preliminary report of experimental and clinical studies. *Proc Staff Meet Mayo Clin* 1941; **16**: 388–95
32. Fogarty TJ, Cranley JJ, Krause RJ, Strasser ES and Hafner CD. A method for extracting arterial emboli and thrombi. *Surg Gynaecol Obstet* 1963; **2**: 241–4
33. Hight DW, Tilney NL and Couch NP. Changing clinical trends in patients with peripheral arterial emboli. *Surgery* 1976; **79**: 172–6
34. Haimovici H. Arterial embolism, myoglobinuria and renal tubular acidosis. *Arch Surg* 1970; **100**: 639–45
35. Dale WA. Differential management of acute peripheral arterial ischaemia. *J Vasc Surg* 1984; **1**: 269–78
36. Cambria RP and Abbott WM. Acute arterial thrombosis of the extremity. *Arch Surg* 1984; **119**: 784–7
37. Jivegard L., Holm J and Schersten T. The outcome in arterial thrombosis misdiagnosed as embolism. *Acta Chir Scand* 1986; **152**: 251–6
38. Scott DJA and Davies AH, Horrocks M and Baird RN. Risk factors in selected patients undergoing femoral embolectomy. *Ann R Coll Surg Engl* 1989; **71**: 229–32
39. Nachbur B. Treatment of acute ischaemia: every general surgeon's business? *Eur J Vasc Surg* 1988; **2**: 281–2
40. Clason AE, Stonebridge PA, Duncan AJ, Nolan B, McL Jenkins A and Ruckley CV. Acute ischaemia of the lower limb: the effect of centralizing vascular surgical services on morbidity and mortality. *Br J. Surg* 1989; **76**: 592–3
41. Hickey NC, Crowson MC and Simms MH. Emergency arterial reconstruction for acute ischaemia. *Br J Surg* 1990; **77**: 680–1
42. Yeager RA, Moneta GL, Taylor LM, Hamre DW, McConnell DB and Porter JM. Surgical management of severe acute lower extremity ischaemia. *J. Vasc Surg* 1992; **15**: 385–93
43. Tawes RL, Harris EJ, Brown WH, Shoor PM, Zimmerman JJ, Sydorak GR, Beare JP, Scribner RG and Fogarty TJ. Arterial thromboembolism: a twenty year perspective. *Arch Surg* 1985; **120**: 595–9
44. Fogarty TJ, Chin AK, Olcott C, Shoor PM, Zimmerman JJ and Garry MT. Combined thrombectomy and dilatation for the treatment of acute lower extremity arterial thrombosis. *J Vasc Surg* 1989; **10**: 530–4
45. White GH, White RA, Kopchok BS and Wislon SE. Angioscopic thromboembolectomy: preliminary observations with a recent technique. *J Vasc Surg* 1988; **7**: 318–25
46. Blaisdell RW, Steel M and Allen RE. Management of acute lower extremity arterial ischaemia due to embolism and thrombosis. *Surgery* 1978; **84**: 822–31
47. Jivegard LE, Arfvidsson B, Holm J and Schersten T. Selective conservative and routine early operative treatment in acute limb ischaemia. *Br J Surg* 1987; **74**: 798–801
48. Cotton LT, Flute PT and Tsapogas MJC. Popliteal artery thrombosis treated with streptokinase. *Lancet* 1962; **ii**: 1081–3
49. McNicol GP and Douglas AS. Treatment of peripheral vascular occlusion by streptokinase perfusion. *Scand J Clin Lab Invest* 1964; suppl 78: 23–9
50. Clark ML, Howell M, Hawkey C, Rees RSO and Stubbs J. Arterial occlusion treated by streptokinase. *Postgrad Med J* 1965; **41**: 96–100

51. Tsapogas MJ. The role of fibrinolysis in the treatment of arterial thrombosis: experimental and clinical aspects. *Ann R Coll Surg Eng* 1964; **34**: 293–313

52. Hirsh J, O'Sullivan EF, Gallus AS and Gilford EJ. Arterial thrombosis in a patient with chronic thrombocytopenia: successful treatment with intra-arterial infusion of streptokinase. *Med J Aust* 1969; **2**: 1304–6

53. Chesterman CN, Nash T and Biggs JC. Small-vessel thrombosis following vascular injury: successful treatment with a low dose intra-arterial infusion of streptokinase. *Br J Surg* 1971; **58**: 582–5

54. Dotter CT, Rosch J and Seaman AJ. Selective clot lysis with low dose streptokinase. Radiology 1974; **111**: 31–7

55. Hess H, Ingrische H, Mietaschk A and Rath H. Local low dose thrombolytic therapy of peripheral arterial occlusions. *N Engl J Med* 1982; **307**: 1627–30

56. Earnshaw JJ. Thrombolytic therapy in the management of acute limb ischaemia. *Br J Surg* 1991; **78**: 261–9

Chapter 2

Metabolic effects of reperfusion injury

I. S. Paterson and C. P. Shearman

Introduction

Tissue ischaemia is a common clinical event with potentially serious consequences and therapy is generally directed at restoring adequate blood flow. Most damage seems to occur upon reperfusion, with the re-introduction of oxygenated blood, and is probably mediated by activated neutrophils. The vascular endothelial cell seems to be the final common target of these mediators and responds by increasing its permeability resulting in tissue oedema. The final injury is thought to be similar in most states of reduced tissue perfusion including limb ischaemia and hypovolaemic shock.

If the mass of ischaemic tissue is large, such as the legs or gastrointestinal tract, then reperfusion injury results in not only local damage but also in systemic manifestations such as the adult respiratory distress syndrome and renal failure[1,2]. In this chapter we discuss the cellular basis of ischaemic reperfusion injury, review the inflammatory mediators and cellular elements involved, put it in the context of thrombolysis and consider potential strategies for treatment.

Reperfusion injury

Two recent observations have been central to improved understanding of ischaemic reperfusion injury. First the re-introduction of oxygenated blood to ischaemic tissue causes considerably more damage than that induced by ischaemia alone. Thus 3 hours of intestinal ischaemia followed by 1 hour of reperfusion causes considerably more injury than 4 hours of ischaemia without reperfusion[3]. Secondly, neutrophils have been demonstrated to be the prime mediator of reperfusion injury. That neutrophils infiltrate infarcted myocardium has been known for many years and was initially thought part of the healing process[4]. In 1983 it was observed that the eventual size of myocardial infarct produced by coronary artery clamping in a dog model could be reduced by prior neutrophil depletion, thus implicating the neutrophil itself as a potentially injurious agent during reperfusion[5]. More recently experimental models have provided an insight into the mechanism of neutrophil mediated injury.

Biochemistry of reperfusion

Under aerobic conditions oxygen undergoes tetravalent reduction by mitochondrial cytochromes with the production of high energy phosphate groups and water (Figure 2.1). However, approximately 2% of oxygen metabolism takes place by univalent reduction outside the mitochondria. This results in the formation of a series of highly reactive and toxic substances including the free radical superoxide (O_2^-), the hydroxyl radical (OH^-) and hydrogen peroxide (H_2O_2)[6-8]. A free radical is an atom or molecule with an unpaired electron in its outer orbital, making it so unstable that it tends to interact with the first atom or molecule with which it comes into contact to achieve a stable energy level. This explains the extreme toxicity of free radicals, and aerobic cells have evolved protective mechanisms to limit such damage. The enzyme superoxide dismutase (SOD) catalyses the reduction of the superoxide radical to hydrogen peroxide, the removal of which is enhanced by another series of enzymes including catalases and peroxidases. There are also antioxidants in the cell cytoplasm such as ascorbic acid, cysteine and reduced

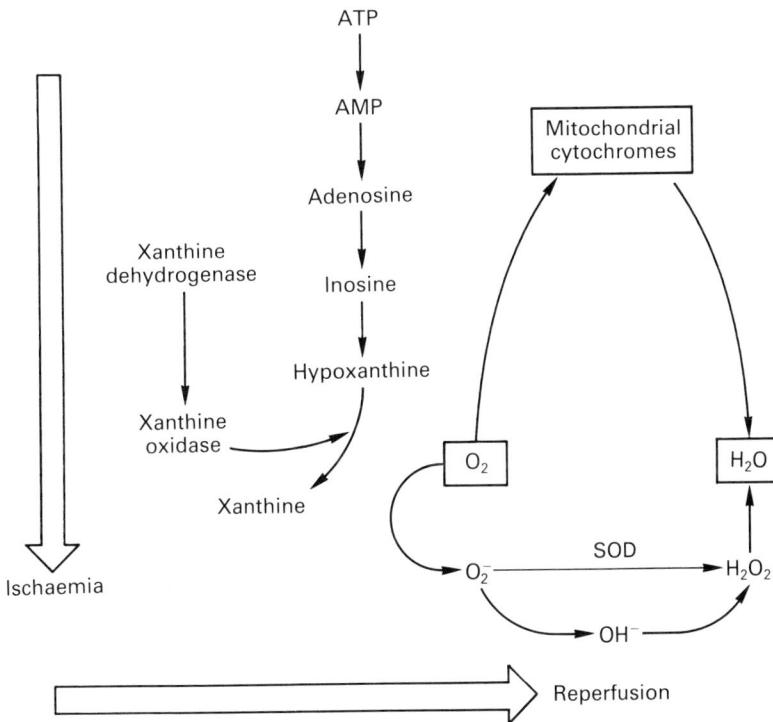

Figure 2.1. Metabolism of oxygen. Aerobic metabolism largely occurs via the cytochrome system within the mitochondria. Ischaemia is associated with the conversion of xanthine dehydrogenase to xanthine oxidase and the build up of hypoxanthine. On reperfusion with oxygen, xanthine oxidase converts the hypoxanthine into xanthine with the production of superoxide (O_2^-). This can be further converted to the hydroxyl radical (OH^-) and hydrogen peroxide (H_2O_2). Superoxide dismutase (SOD) catalyses the rapid removal of superoxide with the formation of water

glutathione which further limit free radical activity. Under normal circumstances few oxygen free radicals will be available to cause tissue damage.

Reperfusion injury is initiated by biochemical events occurring during ischaemia which result in increased generation of highly reactive oxygen metabolites[9]. The first step is depletion of adenosine tri-phosphate (ATP) by its degradation to hypoxanthine. This is normally oxidized by the enzyme xanthine dehydrogenase to xanthine using nicotinamide adenine dinucleotide (NAD) which is converted to NADH. However, during ischaemia xanthine dehydrogenase is converted to xanthine oxidase. This enzymatic conversion is central to the hypothesis of oxygen radical mediated reperfusion injury. Xanthine oxidase has recently been shown to build up during periods of as little as 60 minutes of skeletal muscle tourniquet ischaemia in humans[10].

The second important event in ischaemia is that high levels of hypoxanthine accumulate in tissue. This occurs not only because xanthine dehydrogenase is no longer present but also because xanthine oxidase uses oxygen as its substrate instead of NAD and is therefore unable to capitalize on the conversion of hypoxanthine to xanthine anaerobically. The accumulation of xanthine oxidase and hypoxanthine is not detrimental until reperfusion. When oxygen is re-introduced xanthine oxidase converts hypoxanthine to xanthine with the generation of large amounts of superoxide (Figure 2.1). This burst of superoxide production initiates a cascade of reactions which release other oxygen radicals and hydrogen peroxide within endothelial cells and temporarily overcome the cells' protective mechanisms[11,12].

The importance of oxygen free radicals is emphasized by the protective effect afforded by the infusion of specific scavengers such as superoxide dismutase during reperfusion[13]. The intra-cellular production of these free radical species does not by itself appear to be sufficient to account for the extent of the injury because protection is afforded in all cases of ischaemic reperfusion injury either by prior depletion of circulating neutrophils or by preventing their adherence to vascular endothelium[5,9,14,15]. The important role of the neutrophil is further emphasized by the observation that treatment prior to reperfusion with oxygen free radical inhibitors or during reperfusion with oxygen free radical scavengers prevents neutrophil accumulation in the reperfused tissue. The current hypothesis is that the main pathological effect of the oxygen free radical release is the generation of chemotactic agents leading to the direct migration of activated neutrophils into the reperfused tissue with consequent injury[11,14].

The role of arachidonic acid products

The precise mechanisms linking xanthine oxidase and free radical production to chemotactic activity are not clearly understood. Similarly, the exact identity of the chemotactic agents operative in different settings of ischaemia are unknown, although arachidonic acid products and complement fragments (particularly in myocardial ischaemia) appear to be of key importance[16]. Breakdown products of arachidonic acid (such as thromboxane) are found in high concentrations in plasma soon after the reperfusion of ischaemic tissue. One consequence of free radical release is an increase in intra-cellular free calcium with subsequent activation of plasma membrane phospholipase

A_2 and arachidonic acid breakdown[17]. The inhibition of oxygen free radicals by scavengers prevents the reperfusion induced increase in arachidonic acid metabolites[18]. The pathways for arachidonic acid breakdown are shown in Figure 2.2.

Although there is little evidence to suggest that arachidonic acid metabolites alone can induce endothelial injury independent of neutrophils, there are three mechanisms whereby these products might influence the neutrophil during reperfusion. First, they can act as chemo-attractants and induce neutrophil adhesion to the endothelium. The lip-oxygenase product, leukotriene LTB_4, and the cyclo-oxygenase product, thromboxane A_2, are potent chemoattractants[19,20]. Both are generated in sufficient quantity following ischaemia to induce neutrophil endothelial adhesion and diapedesis. Specific inhibitors of their production following ischaemia attenuate the local reperfusion injury following hind limb tourniquet ischaemia[15]. Secondly, arachidonic acid products may activate neutrophils to produce free radicals and proteolytic enzymes. Leukotriene LTB_4 is a potent stimulant for neutrophil generation of hydrogen peroxide[21] and the hydroxyl ion has been shown to activate neutrophils to induce endothelial permeability *in vitro* and *in vivo*[22]. Thromboxane A_2 also activates neutrophils and mediates their hydrogen peroxide production following ischaemia[23]. Thirdly, thromboxane

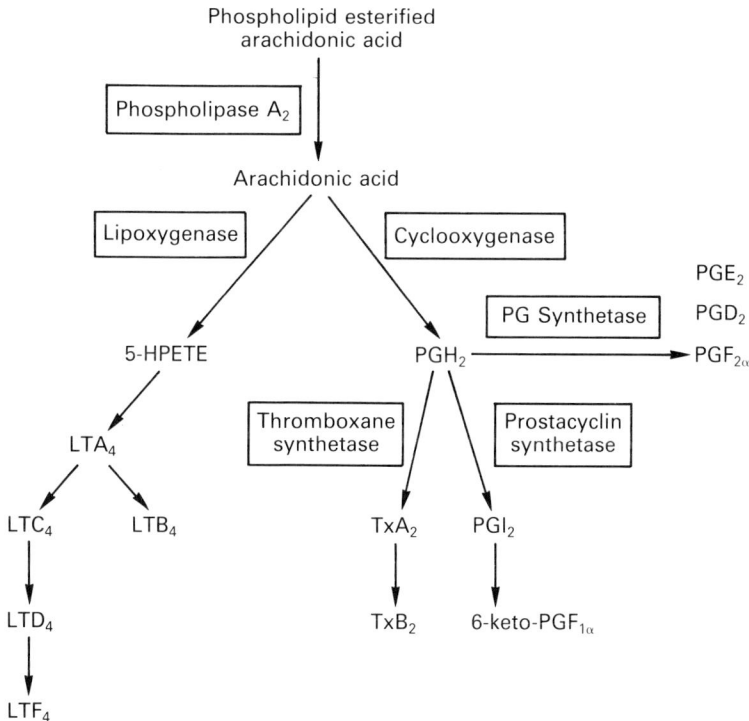

Figure 2.2 The arachidonic acid cascade showing essential products and intermediates. LT = leukotriene, Tx = thromboxane, PG = prostaglandin, 5-HPETE = 5-hydro (pero) xyeicosatetraenoic acid

and the pepto-leukotrienes LTC4 and LTD4 can affect blood flow and therefore tissue perfusion by direct action on the microvasculature. Thromboxane mediated vasoconstriction will exacerbate poor capillary flow after reperfusion[24]. It is not known whether leukotrienes LTC4 and LTD4 are important in ischaemia although they are important vasoconstrictors. Leukotriene LTB4 does not directly affect blood flow[25].

The role of the neutrophil

Neutrophils entering newly reperfused tissue become activated to increase their synthesis of oxygen free radicals and proteolytic enzymes. They also become more adhesive to the endothelium. These activated neutrophils can induce injury by adhering to endothelium in two sites: the pre-capillary sphincter and the post-capillary venule. As activated neutrophils become more viscous they may not be malleable enough to pass through the pre-capillary sphincter. The result is that capillaries become plugged (the no re-flow phenomenon) upon reperfusion with exacerbation of the microvascular injury[26]. Most invading neutrophils adhere to endothelium in the post-capillary venule and induce injury by the secretion of proteolytic enzymes such as elastase[27], probably in conjunction with neutrophil generated oxygen products such as hypochlorous acid and hydrogen peroxide. This results in destruction of essential structural matrix proteins such as elastin and increases microvascular permeability.

Neutrophils must not only be present, but their adherence to endothelium appears to be a prerequisite for vascular injury, creating a microenvironment containing high concentrations of injurious agents. The importance of the neutrophil endothelial interaction following ischaemia has been emphasized by recent work showing that monoclonal antibodies directed against either

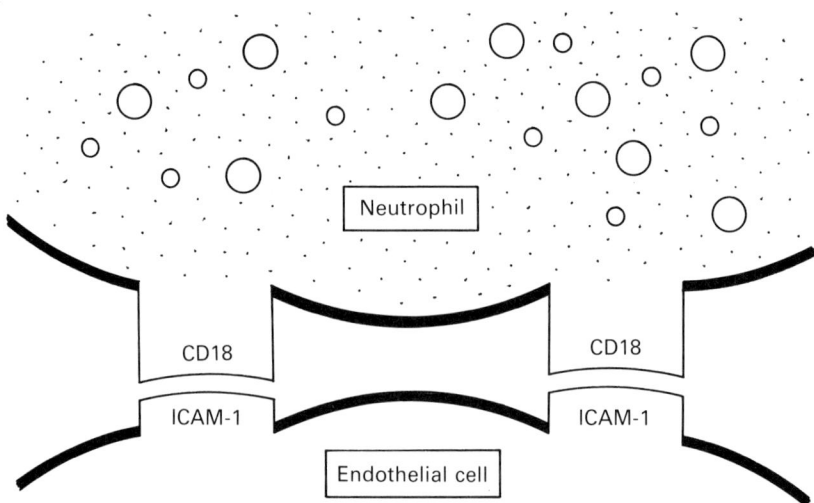

Figure 2.3 Neutrophil, endothelial adhesion molecules

the neutrophil adhesive glycoprotein (CD18 complex) or its endothelial determinant (the inter-cellular adhesion molecule, ICAM-1) are equally effective in preventing reperfusion injury[28,29]. These paired adhesion molecules, CD18/ICAM-1, are the only antigenic determinants of neutrophil endothelial adhesion for which clear roles have been demonstrated in ischaemic reperfusion injury (Figure 2.3).

Remote organ injury following lower limb ischaemia

The reperfusion of a large mass of ischaemic tissue results in a systemic inflammatory reaction and multiple organ dysfunction. The underlying abnormality in all organs is similar to the local reperfusion injury with accumulation of activated neutrophils and an increase in microvascular permeability to protein[1]. After aortic aneurysm repair this occasionally results in adult respiratory distress syndrome type pulmonary oedema, transient increases in plasma creatinine and increases in gut permeability to toxins[30]. Animal studies have demon-strated that the systemic injury is also mediated by the neutrophil[31], but it is not necessary that the neutrophil be activated in the reperfused tissue to cause multiple organ dysfunction. Thus, plasma taken from patients during reperfusion following an aortic aneurysm repair is capable of reproducing a remote microvascular injury in another animal so long as that animal has normal circulating neutrophils[32]. It is likely that additional mediators, possibly cytokines, are generated in the reperfused tissue and these circulate to activate the vascular endothelium of remote organs to attract neutrophils[33].

Reperfusion injury and thrombolysis

It is clear that both the local and systemic reperfusion injuries depend on the mass of ischaemic tissue, the degree of ischaemia and the time before re-oxygenation is achieved. During thrombolysis re-vascularization may occur more slowly than after embolectomy. Selection of patients with less severe ischaemia than those treated surgically may also attenuate the subsequent injury. However, manifestations of a local and systemic reper-fusion injury following lower limb thrombolysis may still be expected. No clinical comparisons are available, but *in vitro* experiments have suggested that local reperfusion injury may be attenuated by thrombolytic agents[34].

We have studied a prospective series of 31 recently thrombosed infra-inguinal long saphenous vein grafts initially inserted for critical ischaemia. The patients all received intra-arterial thrombolytic therapy with re-combinant tissue plasminogen activator (t-PA) at a dose of 0.5 mg/h via a catheter inserted in the contralateral groin 13 ± 6 days after the clinical occlusion of their graft. To try and detect a local reperfusion injury the calf muscle circumference was measured at a constant 10 cm distance distal to the tibial tuberosity on presentation and at 48 hours. All of these patients showed an increase in calf circumference (Figure 2.4) consistent with a local reperfusion injury. Reperfusion injury has previously been suggested as cause for the limb swelling following femoro-popliteal and femoro-distal bypass

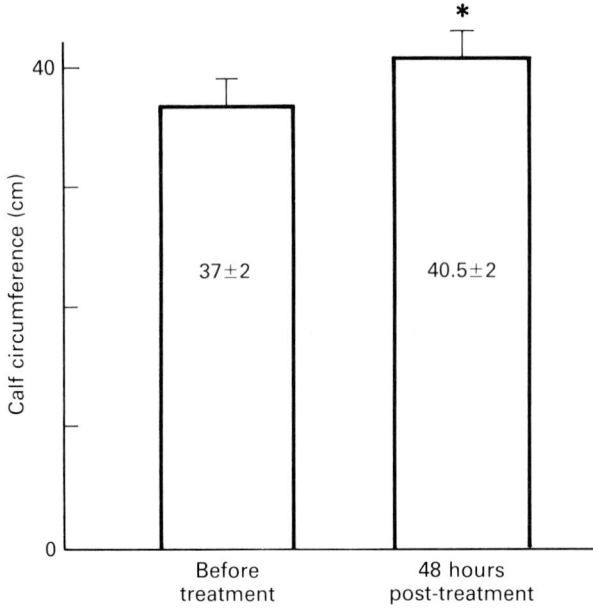

Figure 2.4 Limb swelling after successful thrombolysis of occluded infra-inguinal bypass grafts (* = $P < 0.05$, Rank Sign test)

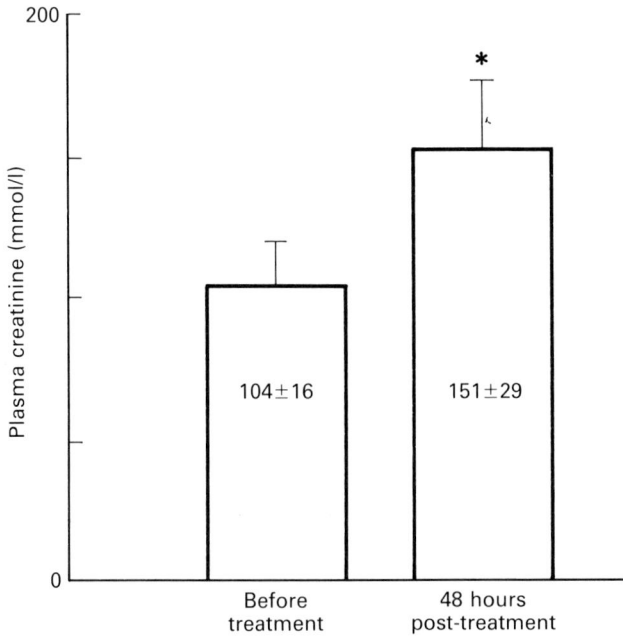

Figure 2.5 Increase in plasma creatinine after successful thrombolysis of occluded infra-inguinal arterial bypass grafts (* = $P < 0.05$, Rank Sign test)

which has been supported by muscle biopsies showing an increased permeability to protein consistent with the mechanism previously described[35]. The contribution of venous and lymphatic damage following groin and popliteal surgery could not, however, be quantified. The increase in calf circumference following reperfusion using thrombolytic therapy is good evidence of the validity of the proposed mechanism.

Previous studies suggest that with regard to the systemic manifestations of reperfusion the lung is disproportionately injured[30]. No patient in our study developed respiratory problems although it is known from animal experiments that this does not preclude an increase in pulmonary microvascular permeability giving rise to subclinical interstitial oedema[18]. The plasma creatinine of our patients rose within the first 48 hours following thrombolytic therapy and this may be a renal manifestation of reperfusion injury (Figure 2.5).

Given the increased interest in accelerated thrombolysis with t-PA, it is likely that patients with a larger mass of more ischaemic tissue will be treated by this technique. Similarly the advent of on-table thrombolysis as an adjunct to catheter thrombectomy may result in the reperfusion of a much larger mass of previously ischaemic tissue than would be achieved by surgery alone. Under these circumstances reperfusion injury may become a limiting factor in the thrombolytic re-vascularization of the ischaemic leg.

Prevention and treatment of reperfusion injury

Experimental evidence from animal models suggests several possibilities. First, substances which scavenge oxygen free radicals or inhibit their production may be effective in limiting the generation of arachidonic acid products during reperfusion. Mannitol, a hydroxyl radical scavenger, reduced thromboxane synthesis and subsequent pulmonary oedema following aneurysm surgery by a mechanism independent of its ability to promote a diuresis[36]. Allopurinol, a xanthine oxidase inhibitor, has been shown to limit reperfusion injury in several animal models but, for maximum efficacy, needs to be administered 12 hours before reperfusion to allow the build up of its active metabolite oxypurinol in the tissues[18,32]. This may limit its use in preventing reperfusion injury in patients undergoing thrombolytic therapy.

In theory, inhibitors of the lipoxygenase or thromboxane synthetase enzyme systems would reduce the generation of chemoattractants, thereby preventing neutrophil migration into reperfused tissue and improving capillary blood flow. Early in vitro studies of a new lipid peroxidase inhibitor provide grounds for optimism[37]. While clinical trials of the more specific inhibitors are awaited, cyclo-oxygenase inhibitors such as ibuprofen and aspirin are potentially hazardous in these clinical settings as they may hinder renal function in addition to their inhibition of prostaglandins. The role of aspirin in peripheral thrombolysis is uncertain though it is beneficial in myocardial thrombolysis (see Chapter 9).

Theoretically a monoclonal antibody directed towards the neutrophil CD18 complex or endothelial ICAM-1 could be used. In vivo studies recently reported suggest that antibody therapy is an effective means of reducing neutrophil accumulation and reperfusion injury.[29] However, it remains to be determined whether they will have clinical benefit.

References

1. Anner H, Kaufman RP, Kobzik L, Valeri CR, Shepro D and Hetchman HB. Pulmonary hypertension and leukosequestration after lower limb ischaemia. *Ann Surg* 1987; **206**: 642–8
2. Schemeling DJ, Caty MG, Oldham KT, Guice KS and Hinshaw DB. Evidence for neutrophil-related acute lung injury after intestinal ischaemia reperfusion. *Surgery* 1989; **106**: 195–202
3. Parks DA and Granger DN. Contributions of ischaemia and reperfusion to mucosal lesion formation. *Am J Physiol* 1986; **250**: G749–53
4. Moon VH. *Shock and Related Capillary Phenomena*. 1938. Oxford University Press; New York, pp. 72–3
5. Romson JL, Hook BG, Kunkel SL, Abrams GD, Schork MA. and Lucchesi BR. Reduction of the extent of ischemic myocardial injury by neutrophil depletion in the dog. *Circulation* 1983; **67**: 1016–23
6. Del Maestro RF. An approach to free radicals in medicine and biology. *Acta Physiol Scand* 1980; (suppl) **492**: 153–68
7. Bulkley GB. The role of oxygen free radicals in human disease processes. *Surgery* 1983: **94**: 407–11
8. McCord JM. The superoxide free radical: its biochemistry and pathophysiology. *Surgery* 1983; **94**: 412–4
9. Granger DN. Role of xanthine oxidase and granulocytes in ischemia reperfusion injury. *Am J Physiol* 1988; **255**: H1269–75
10. Friedl HP, Smith DJ, Till GO, Thomson PD, Louis DS and Ward PA. Ischaemia reperfusion in humans. *Am J Path* 1990; **136**: 491–5
11. McCord JM. Oxygen-derived free radicals: a link between reperfusion injury and inflammation. *Fed Proc* 1987; **46**: 2402–6
12. Ratych RE, Chuknyiska RS and Bulkley GB. The primary localisation of free radical generation after anoxia/reoxygenation in isolated endothelial cells. *Surgery* 1987; **102**: 122–31
13. Granger DN, Rutli G and McCord JM. Superoxide radicals in feline intestinal ischemia. *Gastroenterology* 1981; **81**: 22–9
14. Repine JE, Cheronis JC, Rodell TC, Linas SL and Patt A. Pulmonary oxygen toxicity and ischemia reperfusion injury. A mechanism in common involving xanthine oxidase and neutrophils. *An Rev Respir Dis* 1987; **136**: 483–5
15. Klausner JM, Paterson IS, Valeri CR, Shepro D and Hetchman HB. Limb ischemia-induced increase in permeability is mediated by leukocytes and leukotrienes. *Ann Surg* 1988; **208**: 755–60
16. Pinckard RN, O'Rourke RA, Crawford MH *et al.* Complement localisation and mediation of ischemic injury in baboon myocardium. *J Clin Invest* 1980: **66**: 1050–6
17. Ernster L. Biochemistry of reoxygenation injury. *Crit Care Med* 1988; **16**: 947–53
18. Klausner JM, Paterson IS, Kobzik L, Valeri CR, Shepro D and Hetchman HB. Oxygen free radicals mediate ischemia-induced lung injury. *Surgery* 1989; **104**: 192–9
19. Gimbrome MA, Brock AF and Schafer AI. Leukotriene B$_4$ stimulates polymorphonuclear leukocyte adhesion to cultured vascular endothelial cells. *J Clin Inves* 1984; **74**: 1552–5
20. Spangnuolo PJ, Ellner JJ, Hassid A and Dunn MJ. Thromboxane A$_2$ mediates augmented polymorphonuclear leukocyte adhesiveness. *J Clin Invest* 1986; **66**: 406–414
21. Smedley LA, Tonnesen MG, Sandhaus RA *et al.* Neutrophil mediated injury to endothelial cells. Enhancement by endotoxin and essential role of neutrophil elastase. *J Clin Invest* 1986; **77**: 1233–43
22. Arfors K-E, Lundeberg C, Lindbom L, Lundberg K, Beatty PG and Harlan JM. A monoclonal antibody to the membrane glycoprotein complex CD 18 inhibits polymorphonuclear leukocyte accumulation and plasma leakage *in vivo*. *Blood* 1987; **69**: 338–40

23. Paterson IS, Klausner JM, Goldman G *et al.* Thromboxane mediates the ischaemia-induced neutrophil oxidative burst. *Surgery* 1989; **106**: 224–9
24. Ogletree ML. Overview of physiological and pathological effects of thromboxane A2. *FASEB J* 1987; **46**: 133–8
25. Samuelsson B. Leukotrienes: mediators of immediate hypersensitivity reactions and inflammation. *Science* 1983; **220**: 568–75
26. Engler RL, Dahlgren MD, Morris DD, Peterson MA and Schmid-Schonbein GW. Role of leukocytes in response to acute myocardial ischemia and reflow in dogs. *Am J Physiol* 1986; **251**: H314–22
27. Carden DL and Korthius RJ. Role of neutrophilic elastase in postischemic granulocyte extravasation and microvascular dysfunction in skeletal muscle. *FASEB J* 1990; **49**: A1248
28. Hernandez LA, Grisham MB, Twohig B, Arfors KE and Granger DN. Role of neutrophils in ischemia reperfusion-induced microvascular injury. *Am. J Physiol* 1987; **253**: H699–703
29. Seewaldt-Becker E, Rothlein R and Dammgen JW. In: Springer T, Anderson D, Rosenthal A, Rothlein R (eds) *Leukocyte Adhesion Molecules. Structure, Function and Regulation.* Springer-Verlag, New York, 1990; pp. 138–48
30. Paterson IS, Corson J, McCollum CN, Goldman MD and Middleton MD. Activated neutrophils mediate multiple organ dysfunction following aortic aneurysm repair. *Br J Surg* 1992; **76**: 358–9
31. Klausner JM, Anner H, Paterson IS *et al.* Lower torso ischemia-induced lung injury is leukocyte dependent. *Ann Surg* 1988; **208**: 761–7
32. Paterson IS, Smith FCT, Hamer JD and Shearman CP. Reperfusion plasma contains a neutrophil activator. *Ann Vasc Surg* 1993; **7**: 68–75
33. Stephens KE, Ishizaka A, Larrick JW and Raffin TA. Tumour necrosis factor causes increased pulmonary permeability and oedema. *Am Rev Respir Dis* 1988; **137**: 1364–70
34. Belkin M, Valeri R and Hobson RW. Intra-arterial urokinase increases skeletal muscle viability after acute ischaemia. *J Vasc Surg* 1989; **9**: 161–8
35. Paterson IS, Hanburg A, Browning N, O'Dwyer ST and McCollum CN. Ischaemia and reperfusion as a cause of leg swelling following femoro-popliteal bypass. *Br J Surg* 1991; **78**: 738–9
36. Paterson IS, Klausner JM, Goldman G *et al.* Pulmonary oedema following aneurysm surgery is modified by mannitol. *Ann Surg* 1989; **210**: 796–801
37. Homer-Vanniasinkam S, Hardy SC and Gough MJ. Reversal of the post-ischaemic changes in skeletal muscle blood flow and viability by a novel inhibitor of lipid peroxidation. *Eur J Vasc Surg* 1993; **7**: 41–5

Chapter 3

Intravenous thrombolysis

J. J. Earnshaw

In 1960, following a successful trial of intravenous streptokinase in volunteers with artificially induced forearm venous thrombi, the scene was set for an investigation of the therapeutic potential of thrombolytic therapy. The agent was now 95% pure and allergic reactions infrequent. A series of investigations followed where streptokinase was tested in thrombotic diseases such as myocardial infarction, pulmonary embolism and acute leg ischaemia.

The development of intravenous streptokinase for acute limb ischaemia

Many patients have previously been exposed to streptococcal infections and have antibodies in their serum. It was initially thought therefore that thrombolytic treatment with streptokinase would need to commence with a loading dose to neutralize any pre-existing streptococcal antibodies. After these had been overcome a maintenance infusion would be necessary as streptokinase has a half-life of only 20 minutes. The aim was to induce overwhelming conversion of circulating plasminogen to plasmin and to generate a systemic hyperplasminaemia which would dissolve any abnormal thrombus.

Verstraete and colleagues in Leuven, Belgium investigated the ideal loading dose of streptokinase. It was found that 750 000 u would neutralize all anti-streptococcal antibodies in the serum of 70% of the population. This could be increased to 97% of the population by giving 1.5 million units of streptokinase[1], interestingly the dose presently used for acute myocardial infarction. A maintenance infusion of 100 000 u/h was found to induce the necessary systemic hyperplasminaemia. In initial clinical studies of acute leg ischaemia, a variable loading dose was calculated individually according to measured levels of anti-streptococcal antibodies (the Titrated Initial Dose). However, in the clinical situation, the more complex Titrated Initial Dose had no advantage over a simple standard loading dose of streptokinase[2]. A high initial loading dose (over 2 million units) did not appear to confer any advantage over a loading dose of 500 000 u streptokinase, though with the former method bleeding complications were increased[3]. The standard method therefore became a loading dose of 500 000 u streptokinase, followed by a maintenance infusion of 100 000 u/h.

Table 3.1 Contraindications to intravenous thrombolysis

Absolute
a. Active internal bleeding
b. Recent (within 2 months) stroke or other active intracranial process

Relative
MAJOR:
a. Recent (within 10 days) major surgery, obstetric delivery, organ biopsy, puncture of non-compressible vessel
b. Recent serious gastrointestinal bleeding
c. Recent serious trauma
d. Severe arterial hypertension (>200 mmHg systolic or >110 mmHg diastolic pressure)

MINOR:
a. Recent trauma including cardiopulmonary resuscitation
b. Likelihood of left heart thrombus, e.g. mitral valve disease with atrial fibrillation
c. Bacterial endocarditis
d. Haemostatic defects including those associated with severe hepatic or renal disease
e. Pregnancy
f. Age $>$ 75 years
g. Diabetic haemorrhagic retinopathy

National Institutes of Health Consensus Development Conference. *Ann Int Med* 1980; **93**: 141–4.

The main complications of intravenous streptokinase therapy were allergy and bleeding. Allergy was a common problem induced by impurity of the streptokinase. It was recommended that patients should receive 100 mg intravenous hydrocortisone prior to streptokinase therapy and this decreased allergic reactions. Modern drug purification techniques mean that in most cases this practice is no longer necessary. Major haemorrhage is therefore the most serious complication of intravenous streptokinase. Degradation of plasma fibrinogen produces a hypocoagulable state which can result in haemorrhage from any pre-existing puncture sites or spontaneous bleeding such as intracranial or retroperitoneal haemorrhage. Haemorrhage may be minimized by adhering to guidelines produced by the National Institutes of Health in 1980 which avoids treating high risk patients[4] (Table 3.1). Minimizing the number of invasive procedures and venepuncture sites is also helpful in reducing the risks of intravenous thrombolysis.

Intravenous streptokinase for acute leg ischaemia

The standard regimen for intravenous streptokinase has not evolved much since the 1960s (Table 3.2). Most clinicians still use a loading dose of 250 000–500 000 u which is infused over 90 minutes after initial treatment with hydrocortisone. Subsequently a maintenance infusion of 100 000 u/h is given for a maximum of 72 hours. After this time, the development of antibody resistance to streptokinase will reduce the effectiveness of the drug. In addition, prolonged infusion increases the risk of haemorrhagic complications. Clinical monitoring of the patients is essential. Regular examination of peripheral pulses, Doppler ankle pressures and the degree of distal ischaemia is important. The infusion should be discontinued when the

Table 3.2 Intravenous streptokinase for acute leg ischaemia

Indications	Recent arterial occlusion
	Intra-arterial lysis impossible or unavailable

Avoid invasive arterial or venous punctures within 24 h of treatment

Method	500 000 u streptokinase, infuse over 90 min
	100 000 u/h streptokinase for up to 72 h

Stop infusion after return of pulses and Doppler signals
or if complications
or after 72 h even if no effect

Monitor	Fibrinogen, thrombin clotting time
	Reduce infusion if fibrinogen < 0.5 g/dl

peripheral circulation improves or the peripheral pulses return. Serial measurement of plasma fibrinogen or thrombin clotting time is a useful guide to the possible development of complications and the infusion may be reduced if plasma fibrinogen falls below 0.5–1 g/dl. Measurement of anti-streptococcal antibodies before treatment is unhelpful though there is a relation between the extent of systemic fibrinolysis and the pre-treatment antibody levels.

Results of intravenous thrombolysis

Several authors have published results of patients with acute limb ischaemia treated using intravenous streptokinase[3,5–9] (Table 3.3). In these published reports of 440 cases, a total of 170(39%) had successful lysis. Major haemorrhage was reported in up to 19% of cases, with 4% proving fatal. A further 2% of patients had non-fatal strokes. Stroke is the most feared complication of intravenous streptokinase therapy and is thought to occur in about 3% of patients[10], considerably greater than the 1% rate for peripheral low dose thrombolysis. Overall mortality in these studies ranged from 3% to 16%. A further collected series from Germany included 438 cases and gave similar results with a lysis rate of 46%[11]. The following patients have been shown to have a better chance of successful lysis:

1. Duration of ischaemia less than 72 hours.
2. Emboli compared with thromboses.
3. Distal occlusions compared with proximal.
4. Grafts compared with native vessel occlusions.
5. No neurological deficit prior to treatment.

It is interesting to note that these factors are also applicable to thrombolysis by the low dose intra-arterial route. In a recent report, Fischer describes intravenous streptokinase for 45 patients with recent vascular graft occlusions. Almost 50% had either partial or complete lysis. Results were better for vein than prosthetic grafts[12].

Table 3.3 Results of intravenous thrombolysis with streptokinase in acute leg ischaemia

Author (reference)		Successful lysis		Stroke or haemorrhage		Death	
		No.	%	No.	%	No.	%
Schmutzler, 1968[5]	65	44	68	N/R		N/R	
Amery, 1970[3]	68	21	31	22	32	6	9
LeVeen, 1972[6]	35	16	46	1	3	5	14
Samama, 1973[7]	28	15	54	N/R		1	4
Fiessinger, 1978[8]	194	57	29	18	9	6	3
Earnshaw, 1990[9]	50	17	34	2	4	8	16

N/R = not recorded.

Can results for intravenous thrombolysis be improved?

The most important method of improving outcome with intravenous thrombolysis is careful case selection:

—Treat recent arterial occlusions with no neurological deficit.
—Adhere to the NIH guidelines and exclude high risk cases.
—Avoid unnecessary arterial/venous puncture and invasive procedures.

With knowledge of clinical details as outlined above, the risks for each individual case can be assessed, but treatment of those at high risk is still justified if there is no alternative, providing informed consent is obtained. Modern non-invasive vascular assessment techniques can be used to evaluate patients and are ideal if intravenous thrombolysis is contemplated. Initial assessment with a duplex scan or colour flow Doppler followed by intravenous digital subtraction angiography for confirmation of the arterial occlusion is ideal. Some surgeons avoid treatment of patients with emboli because of the risk of causing further embolization from a cardiac source. Although ECHOcardiography could theoretically identify high risk patients with intracardiac thrombus, clinically this has not been helpful. One-third of all patients with acute leg ischaemia have demonstrable intracardiac thrombus, with approximately equal incidence for both thrombi and emboli. In a study from Nottingham (Table 3.4) there appeared to be no correlation between abnormal ECHOcardiography and stroke during thrombolysis.

Table 3.4 Echocardiography in acute leg ischaemia

	Thrombosis		Embolism	
	No.	%	No.	%
ECHOcardiogram normal	28	74	13	72
ECHOcardiogram abnormal*	10	26	5	28

Nottingham, 1987, unpublished.
* Abnormal ECHOcardiogram = intracardiac thrombus or akinetic segment.

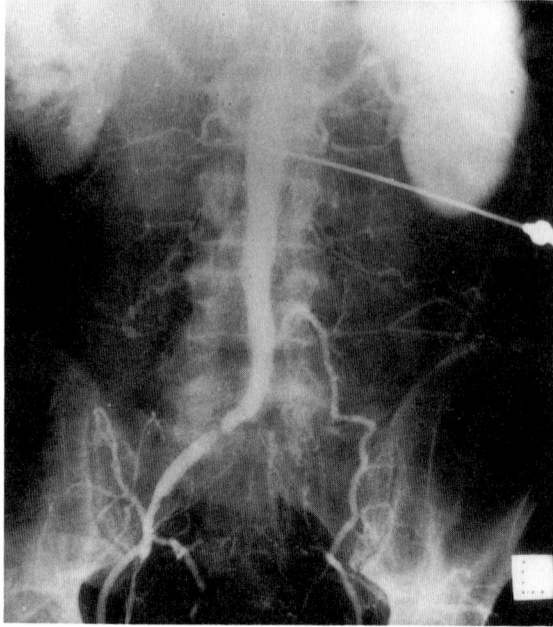

(a)

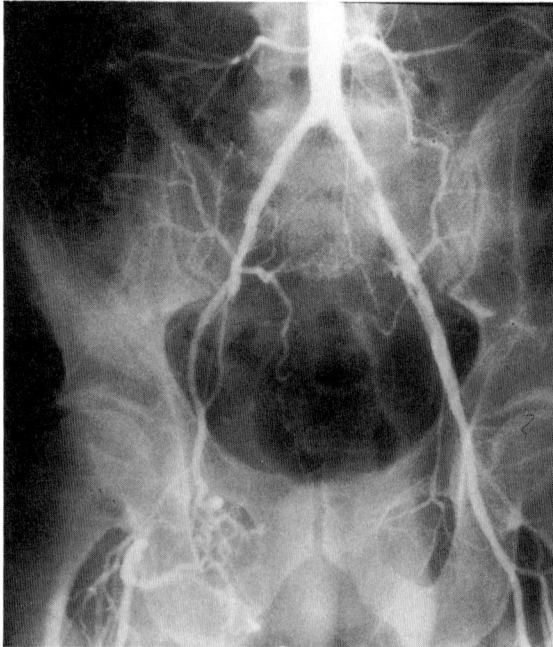

(b)

Figure 3.1 (a) Acute thrombosis of left limb of aorto-bifemoral graft (right limb thrombosed 18 months earlier). (b) Treated with intravenous streptokinase, left femoral pulse restored after 60 hours. Patency maintained with long-term warfarin

(a)

(b)

(c)

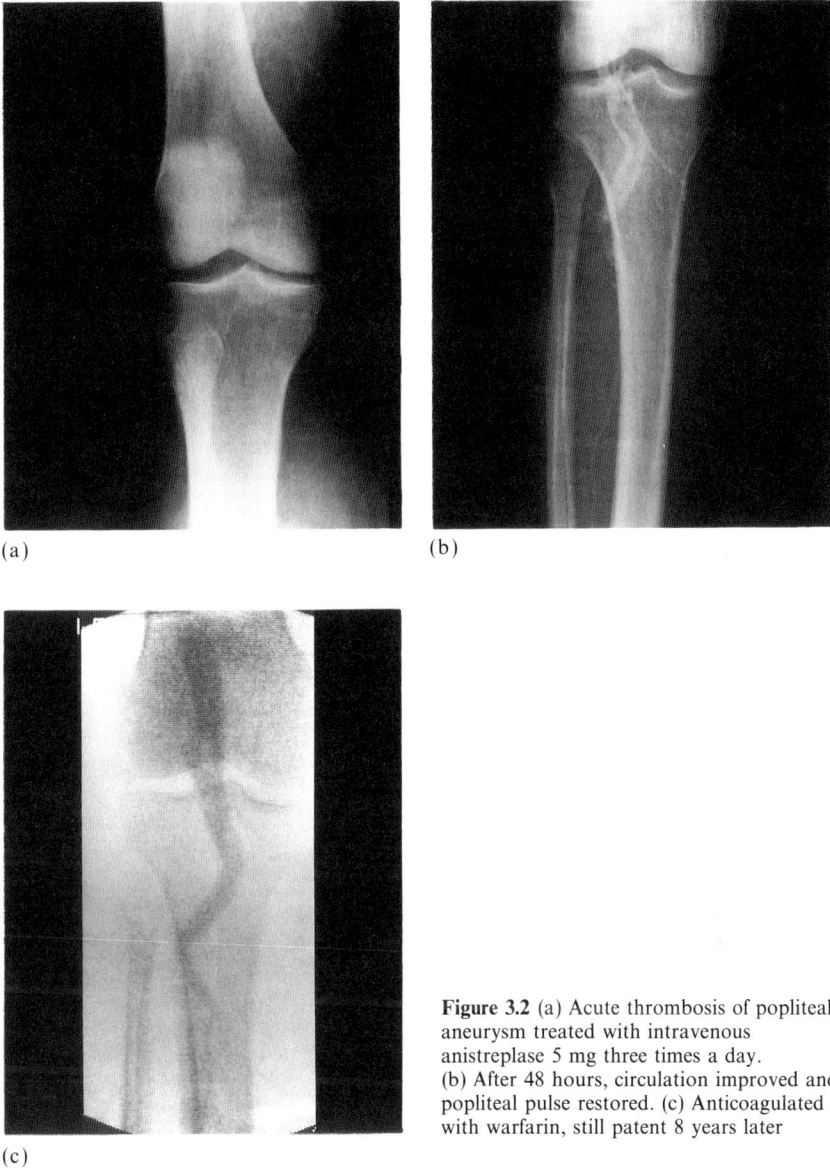

Figure 3.2 (a) Acute thrombosis of popliteal aneurysm treated with intravenous anistreplase 5 mg three times a day. (b) After 48 hours, circulation improved and popliteal pulse restored. (c) Anticoagulated with warfarin, still patent 8 years later

The development of fibrin-specific thrombolytic drugs with the potential to bind to abnormal fibrin offers the possibility of targeted thrombolysis. Two 'fibrin-specific' drugs have recently been developed – anistreplase, an acylated complex of plasminogen and streptokinase (Eminase, SmithKline Beecham Pharmaceuticals) and tissue plasminogen activator (Actilyse, Boehringer Ingelheim). t-PA is produced by vascular endothelium and is responsible for normal plasma fibrinolytic activity (see Chapter 8). Both t-PA and anistreplase can be manufactured in sufficient quantity for clinical use and have been tested intravenously in acute limb ischaemia. Anistreplase has the advantage of a long half-life (40 minutes) and can therefore be administered by intermittent injection, whereas t-PA has a short half-life (2–3 minutes) and is given by infusion. Intravenous injections of 5 mg of anistreplase given 8 hourly to patients with acute limb ischaemia resulted in a lysis rate of less than 30%, with a high incidence of haemorrhagic complications[13]. Similarly, intravenous infusion of t-PA (0.5–10 mg/h) only resulted in a successful lysis rate of 30%[14]. New fibrin-specific thrombolytic agents given intravenously have yet to fulfil their theoretical promise for acute limb ischaemia.

An alternative method of administration of intravenous thrombolytic agents is 'burst therapy' where high doses are given with periods of 'rest' in between to allow at least partial recovery of plasma fibrinogen levels. The aim is to reduce the risk of bleeding without jeopardizing clinical efficacy. Fiessinger used standard streptokinase doses but infused for only 16 hours per day[15]. Persson simply administered 250 000 u streptokinase twice daily[16]. Small studies of both methods yielded inconclusive results.

Intravenous thrombolysis in other conditions

The first condition successfully treated by intravenous thrombolysis was pulmonary embolism. In the first controlled evaluation of thrombolysis which was organized by The National Heart and Lung Institute in the USA, two studies compared heparin and thrombolysis in pulmonary embolism. In the first USPET trial urokinase was shown to speed resolution of pulmonary embolism compared with heparin[17]. In the second study streptokinase and urokinase were compared and found to be equally effective[18]. Despite the power of the studies thrombolysis could only be shown to speed resolution of thrombus and improve pulmonary haemodynamics, but no significant survival advantage could be demonstrated. Similar results have been published using intravenous t-PA[19]. The problem is that pulmonary embolism varies from a minor problem to a severe life-threatening condition. Mild to moderate pulmonary embolism is successfully managed conventionally with heparin (or low molecular weight heparin). The treatment options for severe pulmonary embolism are urgent surgery or thrombolysis. Intravenous thrombolysis may take some time to be effective and time is critical in severe pulmonary embolism. In addition, pulmonary angiography is often required to confirm the diagnosis prior to surgery. It is therefore more logical to give a short catheter directed infusion of a high dose of thrombolytic agent at the time of diagnostic angiography in severe cases. Like peripheral arterial ischaemia, intra-arterial thrombolysis is assuming a more prominent role in acute pulmonary embolism, particularly in severe cases[20].

Myocardial infarction is the commonest arterial thrombotic disease of mankind. Small gains in outcome are of great advantage to the population. Changes in routine management policies have enormous cost implications. Clinicians have responded to this challenge and organized a series of immense randomized trials which have defined optimal treatment for acute myocardial infarction. Since myocardial infarction was shown to be due to coronary artery thrombosis, the potential for thrombolysis has been evident. Initial studies evaluated intra-coronary thrombolysis which was shown to be highly effective. Intravenous thrombolysis for acute myocardial infarction has a lower reperfusion rate but intra-coronary thrombolysis is not applicable as routine management. In randomized trials intravenous thrombolysis was shown to reduce 30-day coronary mortality by up to 25% and has therefore become routine management.

Two aspects of myocardial thrombolysis are of interest for acute limb ischaemia. In the ISIS-2 study of patients with acute myocardial infarction, the addition of aspirin to thrombolytic therapy with streptokinase was beneficial in preventing recurrent infarction and mortality[21]. In ISIS-3, the largest randomized study ever performed including 41 000 patients, there did not appear to be any advantage in using t-PA or anistreplase over streptokinase, a much cheaper alternative[22]. Neither of these studies has been repeated on a similar scale in peripheral arterial thrombolysis, though theoretical implications are discussed in later chapters.

The third indication for intravenous thrombolysis is acute deep vein thrombosis (DVT). This is conventionally treated with heparin to prevent extension of thrombus or pulmonary embolism. Recanalization of the occluded vein often occurs over several months but may result in valve damage and the post-phlebitic limb. The aim of treating DVT with thromb-olysis is to speed recanalization and prevent late development of venous insufficiency. There is evidence of long-term benefit from lysis in a few randomized trials with sufficient follow-up, but all are relatively small. Intravenous thrombolysis exposes the patient to a 1–3% risk of stroke or major haemorrhage, which is probably excessive for most patients with DVT. In addition, many patients develop DVT as a result of surgery, and are therefore not candidates for intravenous thrombolysis. Thrombolysis is useful for patients with extensive ilio-femoral DVT, and is effective if used within 5 days of the onset of symptoms. Its role is now mainly reserved for patients with massive DVT and impending venous gangrene. Catheter-directed infusions of thrombolytic agents are occasionally suggested but have found little role in DVT.

Conclusion

In theory, intravenous thrombolysis should be an ideal treatment for patients with acute limb ischaemia. After a brief non-invasive assessment the ease of administration should have great appeal in the treatment of large numbers of cases. It is a big disappointment that despite major advances in agents and techniques, intravenous thrombolysis does not have a high success rate, which is of the order of 30% even for fibrin-specific agents. It may never be possible to design regimens which are as effective as low dose intra-arterial thrombolysis. This is not illogical as intravenous lysis works best for conditions which present acutely within a few hours, such as myocardial infarction, and have a small volume of thrombus with high local blood flow. Peripheral arterial occlusions often have a large volume of thrombus with low blood flow. Although intra-coronary thrombolysis is not logistically feasible for every patient with myocardial infarction, intra-arterial thrombolysis is a viable alternative for acute limb ischaemia which is a much less common condition.

In a few cases of acute limb ischaemia where percutaneous thrombolysis is impossible or unavailable, intravenous thrombolysis may still be worthwhile. Improvement can be expected in about one-third of patients treated. Though direct comparisons are not available, no advantage has been demonstrated for any of the new fibrin-specific agents over established methods using streptokinase. Careful case selection and attention to detail can optimize results and minimize risks.

References

1. Verstraete M, Vermylen J, Amery A and Vermylen C. Thrombolytic therapy with streptokinase using a standard dosage scheme. *Br Med J* 1966; **1**: 454–6
2. Nilsson IM and Olow B. Fibrinolysis induced by streptokinase in man. *Acta Chir Scand* 1962; **123**: 247–66
3. Amery A, Deloof W, Vermylen J and Verstraete M. Outcome of recent thromboembolic occlusions of limb arteries treated with streptokinase. *Br Med J* 1970; **4**: 639–44
4. National Institutes of Health Consensus Development Conference. Thrombolytic therapy in thrombosis. *Ann Int Med* 1980; **93**: 141–4
5. Schmutzler R. Thrombolytic treatment of acute peripheral arterial and venous occlusions. *Angiologica* 1968; 5: 119–29
6. LeVeen HH and Diaz CA. Venous and arterial occlusive disease treated by enzymatic clot lysis. *Arch Surg* 1972; **105**: 927–35
7. Samama M, Conard J and Bilski-Pasquier G. Streptokinase in peripheral arterial thromboembolism. *Postgrad Med J* 1973; **49** (suppl 5): 91–8
8. Fiessinger J-N, Aiach M, Vayssairat M, Juillet Y, Cormier JM and Houssett E. Traitment thrombolytique des arteriopathies. *Ann Anaesth Franc* 1978; **19**: 739–45
9. Earnshaw JJ, Cosgrove C, Wilkins DC and Bliss BP. Acute limb ischaemia: the place of intravenous streptokinase. *Br J Surg* 1990; **77**: 1136–9
10. Aldrich MS, Sherman SA and Greenberg HS. Cerebrovascular complications of streptokinase infusion. *JAMA* 1985; **253**: 1777–9
11. Hess H. Thrombolytische therapie. In: *Symposion der Deutschen Gesellschaft fur angiologie, Munichen* 1966. Springer-Verlag, Stuttgart: pp. 91–108
12. Fischer M, Heuss F, Hopmeier P *et al.* Results of systemic thrombolysis with streptokinase for recurrent arterial occlusion in the aorto-iliaco-femoral region: a long term trial. *Vasa* 1986; **15**: 61–6
13. Earnshaw JJ, Westby JC, Makin GS and Hopkinson BR. The systemic effect of BRL 26921 during the treatment of acute peripheral arterial occlusions. *Thromb Haemostas* 1986; **55**: 259–62
14. Berridge DC, Gregson RHS, Hopkinson BR and Makin GS. Randomized trial of intra-arterial recombinant tissue plasminogen activator, intravenous recombinant tissue plasminogen activator and intra-arterial streptokinase in peripheral arterial thrombolysis. *Br J Surg* 1990; **78**: 988–95
15. Fiessinger J-N, Aiach M, Brunet G, Cormier JM, LeClerc M and Houssett E. Intermittent treatment with streptokinase in arterial disease of the limbs. *Vasc Surg* 1977; **11**: 384–90
16. Persson AV, Robichaux WT, Jaxheimer EC and Dipronio EM. Burst therapy: a method of administering fibrinolytic agents. *Am J Surg* 1984; **147**: 531–6
17. Urokinase Pulmonary Embolism Trial Study Group. Urokinase pulmonary embolism trial: phase I results. *JAMA* 1970; **214**: 2163–72
18. Urokinase Pulmonary Embolism Trial Study Group. Urokinase-streptokinase pulmonary embolism trial: phase II results. *JAMA* 1974; **229**: 1606–13

19. Goldhaber SZ, Haire WD, Feldstein *et al.* Alteplase versus heparin in acute pulmonary embolism: randomized trial assessing right ventricular function and pulmonary perfusion. *Lancet* 1993; **341**: 507–11

20. Molina JE, Hunter DW, Yedlicka JW and Cerra FB. Thrombolytic therapy for postoperative pulmonary embolism. *Am J Surg* 1992; **163**: 375–80

21. Second International Study of Infarct Survival Collaborative Group. Randomized trial of intravenous streptokinase, oral aspirin, both or neither among 17 187 cases of suspected acute myocardial infarction: ISIS-2 *Lancet* 1988; **ii**: 349–60

22. Third International Study of Infarct Survival Study Group. ISIS-3: a randomized comparison of streptokinase vs. tissue plasminogen activator vs. anistreplase and of aspirin plus heparin vs. aspirin alone among 41 299 cases of suspected myocardial infarction. *Lancet* 1992; **339**: 753–70

Chapter 4

Intra-arterial thrombolysis

A. E. B. Giddings and W. J. Walker

Introduction

The development of intra-arterial thrombolysis

Intra-arterial thrombolysis has been practised for over thirty years but it is only in the last decade that the method has become widely accepted by the majority of interventional radiologists and some vascular surgeons. Following the discovery of streptokinase by Tillett and Garner in 1933[1], it was not until 1959 that its clinical use was suggested[2]. The experience of the 1960s was not encouraging because the high doses and the relative impurity of the agent led to dramatic haemorrhagic and allergic complications. There was no doubt that here was an agent which, for the first time, could remove thrombus which threatened the patient's limb or even his life, but enthusiasm for its local benefits soon became tempered with caution about the systemic risks. The power of local thrombolysis was undoubted, however, and in 1971 Chesterman, Nash and Biggs[3] described the use of low-dose intra-arterial streptokinase in the successful treatment of a small vessel thrombosis following vascular injury. This single case was augmented by Dotter in 1972[4] and again in 1974[5] when he published a detailed description of the method. The techniques were developed in parallel with balloon angioplasty[6]. In 1981 Katzen and van Breda[7] described successful thrombolysis using 5000 u of streptokinase per hour through a 5F catheter and by 1982 Hess[8] was able to report the treatment of 136 patients with successful recanalization in 94, of whom 70 remained patent at 2 weeks.

The Guildford protocol

In Guildford we undertook a study of the method in 1982 and in 1985 published the results of the first British series[9]. There were at that time still problems of selection and control to be overcome but by 1988 greater experience had enabled us to suggest a safer protocol for the use of low-dose intra-arterial streptokinase[10]. The long-term benefits of treatment have now been assessed[11]. Throughout this study we have regarded thrombolysis as a powerful diagnostic and therapeutic tool but one which must be seen as part of an overall strategy for the management of arterial occlusion. Although often an effective and useful treatment, it is not appropriate for every case and does not stand alone (Figure 4.1).

The need for treatment

The need for better methods of treating arterial occlusion is undoubted. In the western world the number of elderly vascular patients continues to rise. By the year 2010 the mean age of the largest population group will be in the sixth decade[12]. Age is a dominant risk factor for vascular disease, as are diabetes mellitus and smoking[13]. All are increasing and there is no prospect that current efforts to alter dietary and smoking habits will have any effect on the prevention of complications from the arterial disease already established in the adult population.

Fortunately for the majority, the increased risk of claudication, which affects 2% of the population in their fifties, 4% in their sixties and 6% in their seventies[14], will threaten an inconvenience to be accepted rather than a severe disability. To avoid the hazards of unnecessary treatment and to spare limited resources for those most in need, at present, in the National Health Service, only patients with severe or progressive claudication are subjected to any radiological or surgical procedure. Even an apparently straightforward and low risk endovascular procedure may go wrong and lead to complex surgery. It is therefore essential that the same criteria should be applied for the selection of patients for both radiological and surgical procedures.

Only a small proportion of those with vascular disease need invasive treatment. Twenty per cent of the population over 75 years of age may have evidence of large vessel peripheral arterial disease[15] and the potential for treatment is considerable, particularly in rich countries with a large medical establishment. There is, at present, a much greater concentration of vascular surgeons and vascular radiologists in the USA than in the UK and rates of surgery and interventional radiology in the two countries reflect that difference. It could be argued that intervention is too frequent in the USA and that 'more does not mean better'; certainly it must be questioned why increasing numbers of angioplasties and bypass operations over the last decade have had no effect on the numbers of amputations for ischaemia[16]. However, the burden of vascular disease is increasing in our ageing populations and valid evidence of the effect of angioplasty and bypass on the quality of life is needed before a judgement about cost and benefit is possible. In the UK it is likely that vascular facilities are relatively underdeveloped and that there is significant potential to reduce rates of premature or unnecessary amputation[17]. The increasing popularity of angioplasty may not reduce the numbers of patients who require vascular surgery[18] but may, at least temporarily, enhance the quality of life for some. Treatment of more minor disease may yield better results and offer less risk but long-term benefits have yet to be proved. It could be argued that in the UK too little financial incentive is available to improve the treatment of more minor but physically incapacitating vascular disease during the most active years of life. While resources are limited it will remain our major challenge to identify those most in need and most likely to benefit.

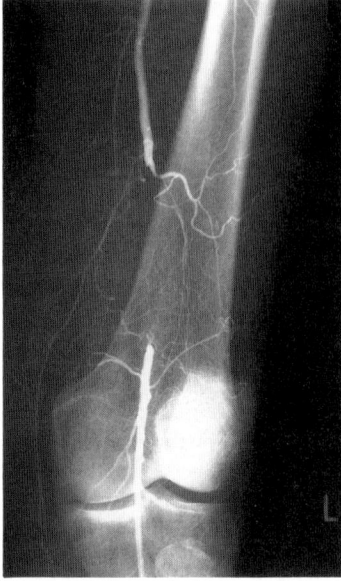

(a)

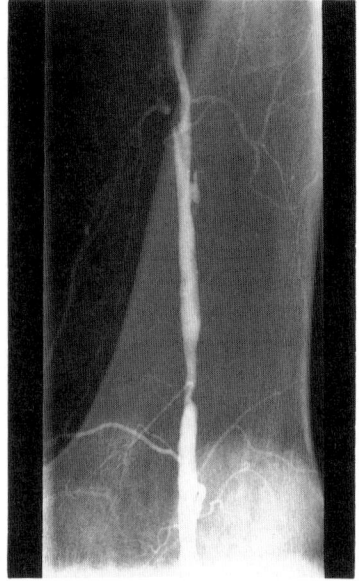

(b)

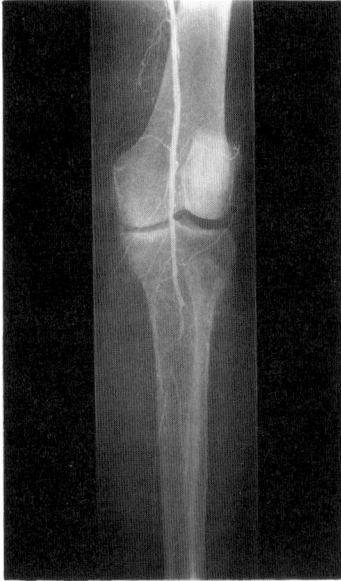

(c)

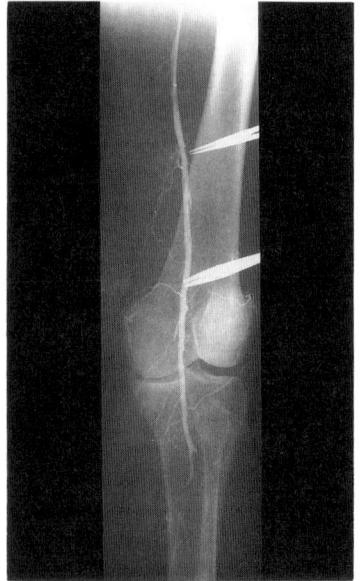

(d)

For patients with critical ischaemia intervention is usually mandatory. Fortunately only 15–20% of patients with intermittent claudication will deteriorate to critical ischaemia, which can be defined by the presence of rest pain, ischaemic ulceration or gangrene. For some, peripheral ischaemia serves to identify them as a person at the extreme of life who is unlikely to

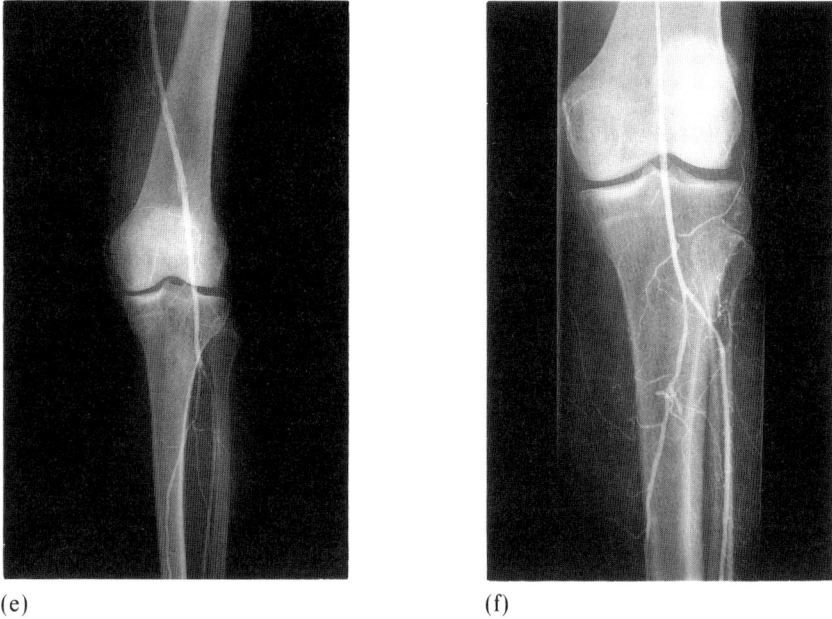

(e)   (f)

Figure 4.1 Thrombolysis does not stand alone. Other procedures such as angioplasty, clot aspiration and surgery may also be required. (a) Chronic left superficial femoral artery occlusion. (b) After initial thrombolysis an atheromatous stricture was revealed. (c) After lysis, the calf vessels were still occluded, possibly due to atheroma or embolism of debris. (d) Angioplasty was performed on the segment marked by the forceps. (e) Further distal thrombolysis only partly cleared the calf vessels. (f) Satisfactory outflow was restored following clot aspiration

survive despite medical treatment. For survivors, however, limb salvage is vital to avoid social handicap and economic dependency, which has been estimated to cost up to £20000 per year[19]. Up to 40% of those presenting with critical ischaemia will be alive in 5 years but many will be amputees and safe thrombolysis has a unique power to save the limb in some of these patients. In the UK critical ischaemia affects about 30 per 100000 of the population, that is at least 5000 patients per year. We estimate that fewer than half of these patients are seen by a specialist vascular surgeon or physician. Only 70% of those admitted will leave hospital with an intact limb. Of the others, half will die in hospital and half will undergo major amputation. Only 20% of the amputees will achieve reasonable mobility with a prosthesis. Thirty per cent will be confined to bed or wheelchair[19].

Most patients with critical ischaemia will present with a gradual deterioration and are best managed by elective investigation. Thrombolysis may sometimes be required to assist angioplasty or reconstruction. Our experience in Guildford shows that about 30% of patients with critical ischaemia present acutely and half of these will be suitable for thrombolysis. They will require urgent intervention and this is our most difficult and critical challenge. In this district of 200000 people, we treat approximately 12 urgent and eight elective patients with thrombolysis each year. To some extent the disadvantages of our small unit are offset by our personal involvement.

Principles in the selection of patients for thrombolysis

Elective investigation: chronic: chronic-on-acute

Patients presenting for elective investigation are usually a more straight-forward challenge than those with urgent problems because they are in a stable condition and have been fully assessed before selection for arteriography. This chronic presentation, however, also includes some in whom the primary event was an acute occlusion and who are therefore 'chronic-on-acute' (Figure 4.2). As Kendrick has shown[20], those who present more than 60 hours after an acute occlusion have a better prognosis and are suitable for elective investigation. Sometimes recent embolism or thrombosis is obvious, or thrombosis has followed elective angioplasty. In these circumstances the indication for thrombolysis is self-evident (Figure 4.3). More commonly arteriography reveals an occlusion but not the cause. Probing with a guidewire may indicate a soft obstruction suggesting recent thrombus suitable for lysis or hard plaque unlikely to respond. There is no certain angiographic sign to distinguish clot which will lyse from mature, resistant thrombus or atheromatous debris and this has led us to approach an obstruction of unknown aetiology by a 'trial of lysis' (Figure 4.4). Ideal positioning of the catheter is required and a check film after 12 hours of infusion. If there is no improvement the infusion must be discontinued since higher doses and a longer duration are unlikely to succeed and will certainly increase the risk of haemorrhage. Some improvement justifies repositioning the catheter for a further trial. Resistant debris will require removal by clot suction or surgery (Figure 4.5).

Urgent investigation: acute: acute-on-chronic

Assessment of these patients is much more difficult because we know less about them; their condition is often unstable and time is short. Severe ischaemia demands relief within 6, or at most 12, hours. Studies of embolectomy have shown that between 12 and 60 hours after a major occlusion, surgery is both ineffective and dangerous, and the patient is best managed by anticoagulation and medical support[21]. After 60 hours the outlook improves and elective investigation is appropriate. Both time and severity are therefore important in the assessment of the urgent case.

The changing pattern of limb ischaemia

The aim of treatment is to save the limbs of those who are likely to survive. For patients with emboli less than 6 hours old, severe ischaemia and a neurosensory deficit, urgent surgery remains ideal, particularly when guided by arteriography. At the other end of the spectrum there will be some in whom necrosis is advanced or inevitable or in whom overwhelming disability makes palliative care appropriate.

Between these extremes are the majority of patients in whom the ischaemia is acute-on-chronic and arterial thrombosis is more likely than cardiac embolism. The declining incidence of rheumatic heart disease and better cardiac care have significantly altered the presentation of acute limb ischaemia over the past 40 years. With the introduction of the Fogarty

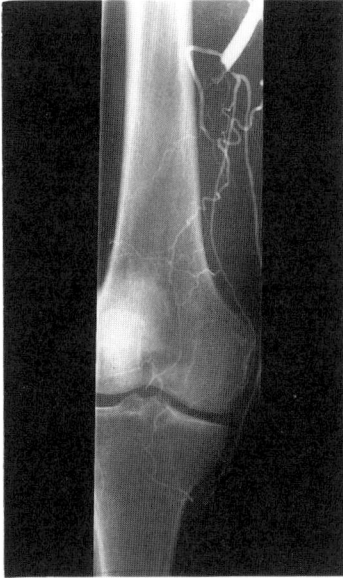

(a)

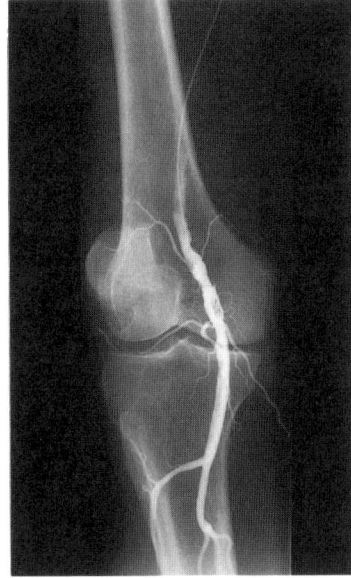

(b)

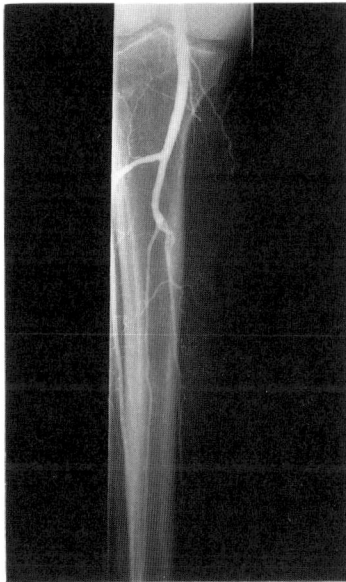

(c)

Figure 4.2 Chronic-on-acute ischaemia.
(a) Diagnostic angiogram several weeks after
episode of acute ischaemia suggesting
embolism. (b) Thrombolysis revealed
occlusion to be due to thrombosis in
atherosclerotic artery. (c) Thrombolysis
followed by angioplasty produced a good
result

balloon catheter in 1963[22] the extraction of arterial emboli and thrombi
from normal vessels was immediately advanced. Even now it remains the
definitive treatment for recent cardiac embolism and acute white leg, but
only 15% of urgent patients now suffer from systemic embolism. Arterial
thrombosis is now the chief cause of the ischaemic limb, particularly when
the presentation is acute-on-chronic rather than acute.

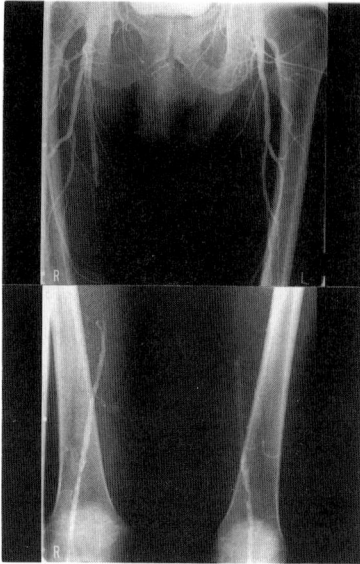

(a)

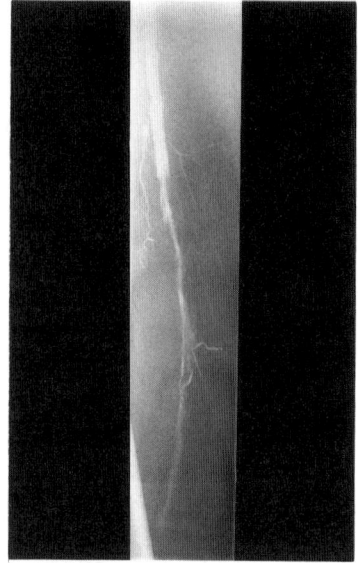

(b)

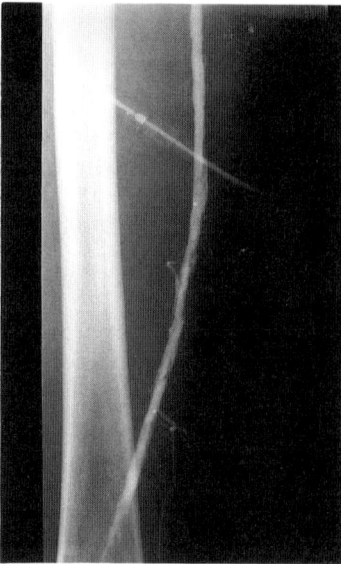

(c)

Figure 4.3 Early re-thrombosis after
successful angioplasty is an excellent
indication for thrombolysis. A good result
can be expected if there was good run off
after the initial angioplasty. (a) Early
re-thrombosis of right superficial femoral
artery angioplasty. (b) Thrombolysis of
angioplasty segment. (c) Successful outcome
after thrombolysis and further angioplasty

The pathology, the best management and the outcome are significantly
different for patients with cardiac embolism compared to native vessel or
graft thrombosis. The risk of embolism is to life, with a 30-day mortality
rate of 17% and an amputation rate of about 13%, whereas for thrombosis
mortality is less at 9% but the risk of amputation much higher at 28%[23].
Although for all patients mortality has declined as medical management of

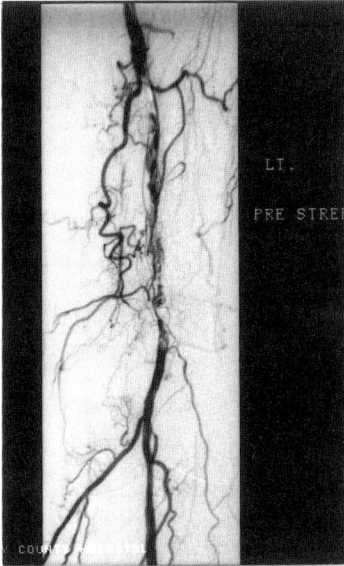

(a)

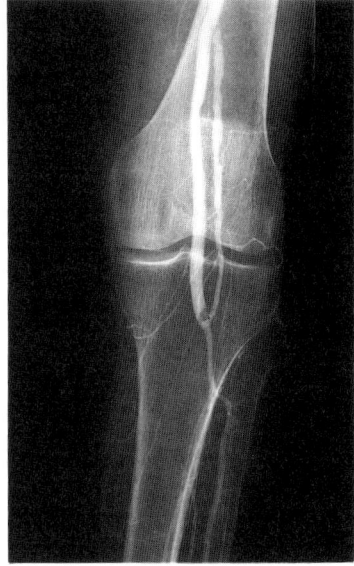

(b)

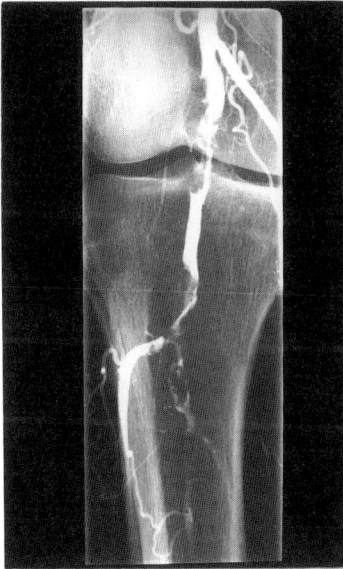

(c)

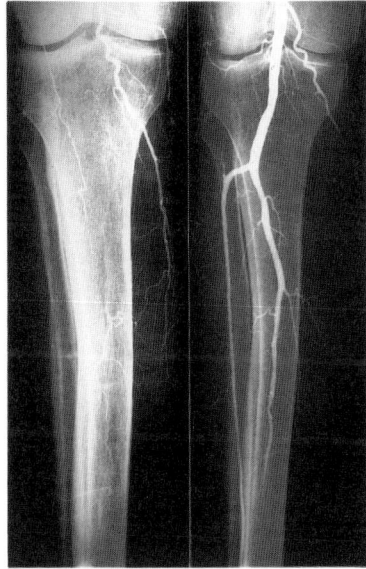

(d)

Figure 4.4 Angiographic appearances may be deceptive and often a trial of lysis is justified. (a) A long irregular femoro-popliteal occlusion most likely due to severe atheroma. Successful thrombolysis unlikely. (b) Distal filling defect after successful lysis of a femoro-popliteal graft. Looked like embolus but was actually fibrous hyperplasia requiring surgery. (c) Appearances suggested embolism but the lesions were atheromatous. (d) Failed thrombolysis of popliteal occlusion (left). After clot aspiration the embolus was removed and patency restored (right)

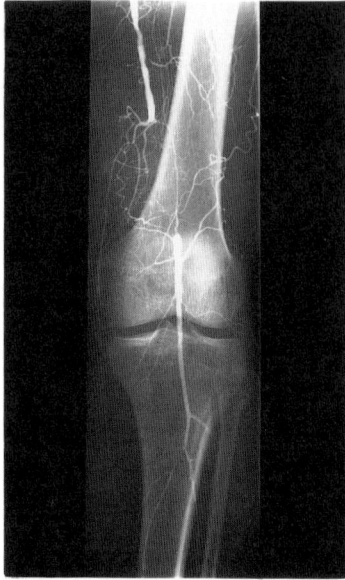

(a)

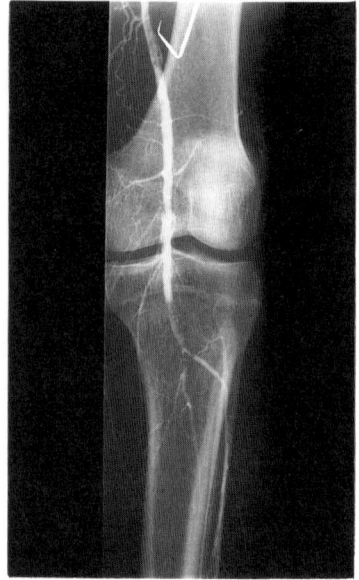

(b)

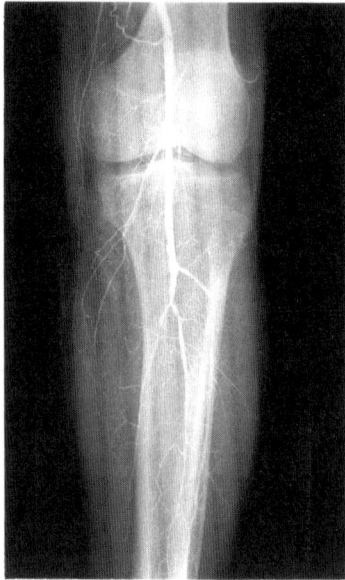

Figure 4.5 (a) Left superficial femoral artery occlusion treated by primary angioplasty. (b) Distal embolization occluded the popliteal artery. A trial of lysis was unsuccessful. (c) Surgery was required to remove the atheromatous debris; operative angiogram shows successful clearance followed by vein patch repair

(c)

the heart and circulation has improved, that decline has been by only 5% since the introduction of balloon embolectomy, probably because there are now more elderly patients at risk. The effect of balloon embolectomy on long-term limb salvage has also been small[24]. The dramatic benefit from appropriate use of balloon embolectomy is self-evident but is now less often required and blind embolectomy is likely to be the wrong treatment for most patients with acute-on-chronic ischaemia. Medical support and anti-coagulation with heparin will improve the outcome for life and limb with minimal risk; it is certainly to be preferred when limb viability is in doubt[25,26]. Safe thrombolysis offers the prospect of further improvement but it is essential to minimize risk.

Contra-indications to thrombolysis: absolute; relative

Absolute contra-indications may be thought of as circumstances in which thrombolysis is either inappropriate or dangerous. It is certainly in-appropriate where recent ilio-femoral embolism and a neurosensory deficit demand immediate surgical embolectomy or where tissue loss is established. To avoid certain danger, especially stroke, it is necessary to exclude any patient known to have a bleeding tendency and particularly anyone who has suffered a stroke within the preceding 2 months. While the risk of stroke is small[27] when a correct protocol is followed, probably about 1%, it is a major problem because the management of the limb and the stroke are conflicting and because stroke so often leads to death or expensive and degrading disability in those who survive.

Relative contra-indications include recent previous treatment with strepto-kinase and the post-operative patient in whom the benefits of lysis must be balanced against the risk of renewed bleeding from surgical incisions or vessel punctures. It is also unwise in the puerperium, or when there is peptic ulceration, liver disease, portal hypertension, thrombocytopenia, bacterial endocarditis, acute pancreatitis and severe renal failure or after traumatic resuscitation (see Chapter 3). These relative contra-indications are usually given for systemic dosages and may be cautiously relaxed for low-dose peripheral infusions. We generally also avoid lysis in the upper limb since the vessels are narrow, tortuous and prone to spasm (Figure 4.6(a)). Additionally there is a theoretical risk that pericatheter thrombosis may occur in the innominate or subclavian arteries and lead to cerebral embolism, but documented instances are very rare using modern techniques. Lysis should usually be avoided in a Dacron® (E.I. Dupont de Nemour Incor-porated) graft implanted in the retroperitoneal space since bleeding through the weave of the graft may occur even when it appears well incorporated into surrounding tissues; such bleeding is dangerously occult.

The relative contra-indication of allergy may be overcome by the use of alteplase (tissue plasminogen activator; t-PA) (Actilyse®, Boehringer Ingel-heim) although this increases the cost. At present 250 000 iu of streptokinase costs under £20 and 20 mg of alteplase costs £175. Relative contra-indications should include confusion and restlessness since a co-operative patient is necessary for the safe use of intra-arterial catheters over several hours. It would be very unwise to attempt thrombolysis if experienced medical and nursing staff were not readily available to place the catheter, monitor the infusion and provide complete radiological, surgical and nursing care.

Using a licensed drug for an unlicensed purpose

As neither streptokinase nor t-PA is licensed for intra-arterial use under the Medicines Act of 1968, while doctors are free to use them, they must be

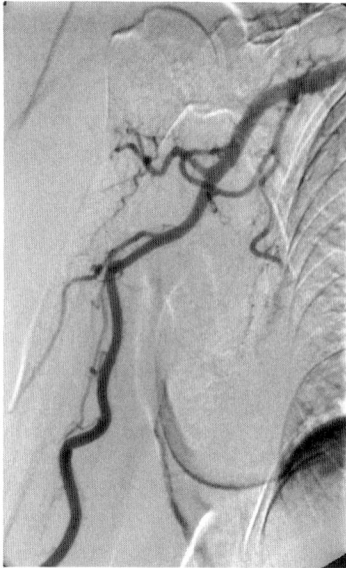

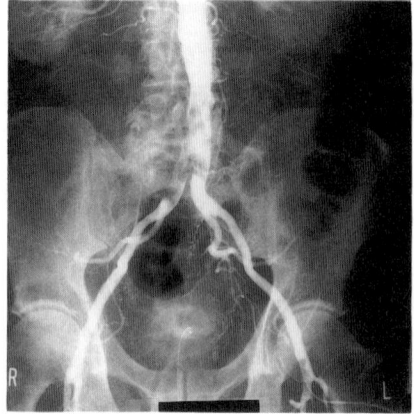

(a)

(b)

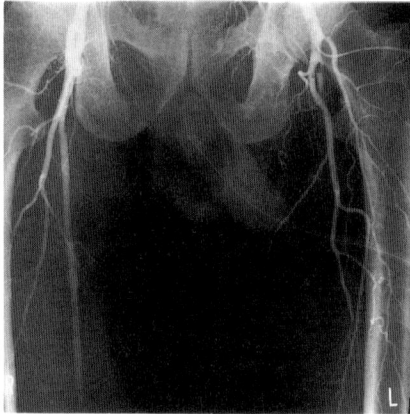

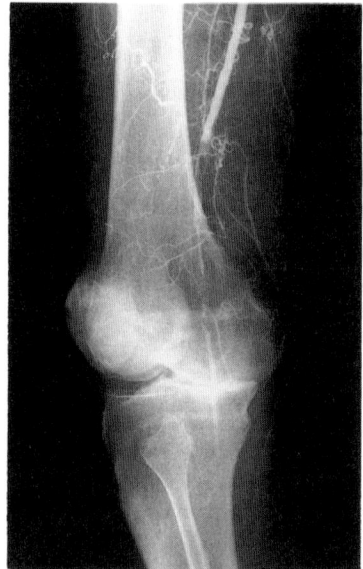

(c)   (d)

Figure 4.6 Relative contraindications to thrombolysis. (a) Tortuous upper limb arteries.
(b)–(d) Multiple emboli in the same patient. (b) Aortic saddle embolus with embolus in left
common femoral artery. (c) Embolus obstructing left superficial femoral artery. (d) Embolic
occlusion of right popliteal artery

particularly careful to take 'reasonable care' and 'to act in a way consistent
with the practice of a responsible body of their peers of similar professional
standing'[28]. Irregular techniques would risk allegations of negligence,
whereas following a correct protocol helps to provide safety for the patient
and some protection for the doctor.

Assessment of the patient

History: examination: investigation

These are the tools with which we build a complete understanding of the heart and circulation before assessing the importance of a particular lesion.

History

The more you know, the better. Question whether the patient is normally active and independent or whether they have already adapted to sedentary dependence? And what of the limb? Systematic recording of the nature and duration of the presenting complaint is vital, particularly to distinguish an acute from an acute-on-chronic presentation. Acute ischaemia is often a memorable and dramatic event (though it may have been several weeks ago) and sudden embolism is sometimes easily distinguished from a thrombosis due to progressive stricture. The patient's general medical condition must also be assessed as peripheral ischaemia may be secondary to low cardiac output, 'pump failure'. Atrial fibrillation, palpitations, angina, fatigue or breathlessness may indicate serious heart disease which is now exposing a previously unrecognized obstruction. Embolism may follow a change in cardiac rhythm. Thrombosis may follow diuretic or diabetic dehydration. Heavy smoking or respiratory disease make haemoconcentration and enhanced viscosity likely. Previous claudication may indicate an established obstruction at one level, which is now complicated by a second, acute occlusion at another site. Careful analysis of the history, supported where possible by previous records, can help to avoid treatment of the wrong lesion.

The effects of ischaemia are first seen in tissues which have the highest metabolic demand, nerve and muscle. The history of pain is particularly important. The muscle pain of claudication has a reproducible pattern on exertion but the rest pain of severe ischaemia is intractable and associated with numbness and paraesthesia. It may be eased by dependency, but this will encourage oedema, venous stasis and thrombosis, all leading to reduced arterial perfusion. Ulceration and infection enhance demand and must be noted. Current medication and any history of allergy must be clearly recorded.

Examination

The general medical state should be assessed first, including pulse rate, rhythm and pressure. Arrhythmia and failure of the heart should be recorded especially noting apex rate, venous pressure, oedema and signs of pulmonary congestion. Peripheral pulses and palpable aneurysms should be described and where pulses are impalpable the arteries should be interrogated using a hand-held Doppler probe. Systolic pressure may then be recorded in impalpable arteries and patency established even in vessels with very poor perfusion. Doppler studies in the dependent limb, assisted by squeezing the muscles or pulse generated run-off techniques, may be better than arteriography at showing patent small arteries[29].

A femoral pulse of variable volume suggests severe cardiac disease or an incomplete obstruction. Patency indicates the potential for improvement. In the symptomatic limb, acute arterial occlusion will be seen as a pale, cool limb with empty veins and a distal neurosensory loss, whereas more prolonged ischaemia and dependency, due to rest pain, will lead to oedema and venous congestion. The strongest pulse (a water hammer pulse) may be felt proximal to a recent embolic occlusion, usually just above the femoral bifurcation. Doppler examination confirms that the vigorous pulse is associated with little or no forward flow. Buerger's sign should always be sought. The pallor on elevation is apparent after 2 or 3 minutes even in a congested limb and the slowly returning rubor of dependency clinches the diagnosis and gives an indication of the arterial inflow. The rubor of ischaemia is cold to the touch. It is a reliable test which may also reveal unsuspected ischaemia in the contra-lateral limb. The blue limb of major venous thrombosis is usually warm. Do not forget to listen to the veins with the Doppler, since patent femoral and popliteal veins may be confirmed on compression of the calf muscle. This is a reassuring sign as thrombosis of the popliteal vein, particularly when secondary to arterial occlusion, is a sign of a very poor outlook for the leg. The presence of ulcers, gravitational skin damage, gangrene and inflammation should also be recorded, not overlooking the heel. The level of sensory loss, motor paralysis or rigor should be noted so that improvement or deterioration can be identified. Tissue crepitus caused by infection with gas-forming organisms demands urgent diagnosis. It is due either to gas gangrene from *Clostridium welchii* or the much more common and benign condition of non-clostridial gas gangrene, sometimes seen in the diabetic[30].

Investigation

Most patients with ischaemia have general medical problems and baseline investigations should include a chest X-ray, electrocardiogram, blood count, film and sedimentation rate or plasma viscosity, serum creatinine, electrolytes, glucose, proteins, thyroid function tests and urinalysis. Other tests such as digoxin levels, arterial blood gases and blood cultures may be indicated in selected patients, and before thrombolysis preliminary estimation of fibrinogen and clotting screen are essential.

Screening for thrombophilia may be desirable although it is usually reserved for patients with recurrent venous thrombosis. If thrombophilia affecting arteries is suspected, screening need not include protein C or antithrombin III deficiencies but protein S deficiency and lupus inhibitor/anticardiolipin antibodies may be important.

The acquisition of all this data is not an end in itself but is used to decide how best to treat the patient who presents with an ischaemic limb although the dominant problem may be a failing heart, obstruction in a large vessel, thrombosis in small vessels, polycythaemia, venous obstruction or a combination of several of these factors. Careful diagnosis is essential before treatment is decided.

The technique of thrombolysis

Informed consent

Before premedication or sedation are given, the patient and his nearest relatives should understand as far as possible the condition to be treated and any potential hazards. It is neither necessary nor desirable to go into much technical detail but it is vital that they appreciate the serious nature of limb ischaemia, the possibility of limb loss and the general medical risks. It should also be understood that arteriography, thrombolysis and surgery may all be required as part of an overall treatment plan and that success cannot be guaranteed. Alternative methods of managing the situation should be referred to and the reasons for recommending thrombolysis should be explained. The patient and his family should feel that they have had the opportunity to be involved in these decisions. Some prefer to accept advice with minimal explanation but we must always remember that it is the patient and family who must live with the consequences. Surprisingly, in most instances, it is quite possible to set out these strategic aims in a few simple sentences.

It is also necessary to describe what will actually happen and what may go wrong. The patient may be nursed in an intensive care unit and be required to lie flat for a period of 12–24 hours. Pain from arteriography and thrombolysis is now unusual but the prolonged immobility is uncomfortable and inconvenient. Keeping the patient 'nil by mouth' in case surgery is required is also a trial. The hazard of bleeding must be specifically explained, since even in the best circumstances serious bleeding may occur in 5% of cases. It is not our practice to discuss the smaller risk of stroke (1%) since this is a sporadic risk which our protocol is designed to avoid and we consider that the anxiety caused to patients and their families during treatment would be unreasonable. That risk, however, must never be forgotten by the medical and nursing staff in their care of the patient.

In our hospital the patient is asked to sign a consent form which describes the procedure and its possible complications in some detail. No written record can be a substitute for a clear and sympathetic explanation but it serves as a reminder of the main points to be covered and is a formal record of that contact. Particularly in urgent circumstances neither patients nor their relatives are likely to understand or retain all that is said and continued explanation by medical and nursing staff is usual and helpful as the treatment proceeds. Time spent in explanation is rarely wasted and the risk of misunderstandings, which are often the cause of litigation, is thereby reduced.

Preparation of the patient

This should be as for any surgical operation, keeping the patient 'nil by mouth', using a theatre gown and stretcher canvas and preparing the operative field by antiseptic cleaning and shaving where appropriate. A sheepskin over the canvas helps patients to be comfortable while having to lie still for several hours and a bed cradle and soft supports, such as foam ring 'doughnuts' for the legs are vital to protect ischaemic feet, especially the heels, from any avoidable pressure. A pillow placed under the legs to support the heels is an alternative.

Blood should have been taken for fibrinogen and an initial clotting profile and the results should be recorded in the notes. A nurse, who understands what is to happen, should accompany the patient to the radiology department and hand over to another member of the nursing staff there. They should explain the unfamiliar environment to the patient and maintain continuous observation. Nursing staff must understand the reasons for contra-lateral punctures and be quite sure which limb is being treated.

Sedation and analgesia

All patients should be sedated for the procedure. Local anaesthetic, intravenous sedation and intravenous analgesia are required. Reliable intravenous access is required to avoid bleeding following intramuscular injections. There may be pain from the ischaemic limb. Puncture of the groin is uncomfortable even following administration of a local anaesthetic, and patients are often extremely apprehensive in the bewildering atmosphere of a modern radiological suite. Painful stimuli, enhanced by anxiety, can give rise to hypertensive episodes and restlessness which may hamper the procedure. Particularly uncomfortable moments should be covered by analgesia first. Manipulation of catheters in the groin may cause pain as the effect of the local anaesthetic wears off and the injection of iodine-containing contrast media for the arteriogram may be painful. General anaesthesia is rarely required but the assistance of an anaesthetist is invaluable and the recommendation of the Joint Working Party on Sedation and Anaesthesia[31] should be considered.

In our department we use a mixture of midazolam 10 mg in 2 ml, fentanyl 100 μg in 2 ml and metoclopramide 10 mg in 2 ml, added to 10 ml of 0.9% normal saline, the total volume being 16 ml. This sedative and analgesic mixture is then administered in 3 or 4 ml aliquots to give the level of analgesia required. The patient should be monitored by regular observation of pulse, blood pressure and respiratory rate as well as pulse oximetry, as if unconscious. Facilities for resuscitation including oxygen and suction must be readily available to deal with hypotension, bradycardia or respiratory depression, although in our experience they are seldom needed.

Antibiotics

Thrombolysis is an invasive vascular operation and arterial catheters are often in place for many hours. Prophylaxis with a broad-spectrum antibiotic such as cephazolin 1 g, given before the arterial puncture, is recommended. A clean, sterile operative field is essential and especially important if a graft is punctured directly or if the patient has any artificial prosthesis such as a heart valve or arterial graft.

Femoral artery puncture

A track should be made through tissue infiltrated with local anaesthetic after a small skin incision with a scalpel. This incision allows easy manipulation of the catheter and drainage of blood to minimize haematoma. The artery should be punctured cleanly below the inguinal ligament where digital pressure can control the puncture site. Above the ligament the artery often courses posteriorly around the pelvic brim making arterial cannulation less certain, significantly increasing the risk of occult bleeding and making direct pressure more difficult to apply. The initial approach is usually made from the contra-lateral groin. An anterior, single wall puncture technique is preferred as this minimizes the risk of bleeding. The classic Seldinger double wall puncture and withdrawal of the cannula into the arterial lumen is also acceptable.

The contra-lateral approach.

This is the only approach for thrombus in the iliac, common femoral or proximal superficial femoral arteries. There are several other advantages which are:

1. A full diagnostic arteriogram can be carried out prior to the thrombolytic infusion. This is particularly important in systemic embolism where thrombus may be seen at several levels and also found in the asymptomatic limb (Fig. 4.6(b)–(d)). The presence of occlusive disease and aneurysms at several sites may be noted and all run-off vessels below the obstruction should be demonstrated.
2. With a puncture in the proximal common femoral artery the catheter is more stable and the artery is more easily compressed to control oozing around the catheter site. This is an almost inevitable accompaniment of the procedure.
3. The puncture itself is retrograde and easier than an antegrade puncture. A single wall puncture is more likely to be achieved at the first attempt.
4. Once the catheter has passed into the contra-lateral limb it can be left in place not only for the infusion of thrombolytic agents but also for radiological contrast, heparin and for subsequent diagnosis and treatment. It is particularly useful for intra-operative arteriography.
5. When removing the catheter and compressing the artery there is no reduction in the arterial supply to the treated leg.

The contra-lateral approach, however, does require technical skill, particularly in tortuous or stenotic vessels. It also carries specific disadvantages which are:

1. Angioplasty of lesions below the inguinal ligament is more difficult from the contra-lateral groin. Where angioplasty is required an additional puncture of the ipsi-lateral common femoral artery is usually necessary.
2. Clot suction techniques cannot be applied without ipsi-lateral puncture.
3. If ipsi-lateral puncture is also required then there will be two puncture sites. This is not usually a serious disadvantage and often it is useful to leave the contra-lateral catheter in place after removal of the ipsi-lateral catheter so that completion arteriography can be carried out.
4. There is a greater length of catheter within the patient which may increase the risk of pericatheter thrombosis; this complication is rare with good pericatheter flow. It is essential that small catheters are used and that any strictures through which the catheter has to pass are dilated before carrying out prolonged infusion. Following these principles should make the use of concomitant heparin unnecessary.

The ipsi-lateral approach

This is the optimal approach for thrombus in the popliteal and tibial arteries. It provides the best direct access for angioplasty and clot suction and the least risk of pericatheter thrombosis but carries the disadvantage that arteriography through the catheter is incomplete. Antegrade puncture is considerably more difficult and multiple punctures are necessary in some cases. The puncture site may be above the inguinal ligament and be difficult to compress, particularly in obese patients.

Controlling bleeding around the catheter

An oblique, clean arterial puncture through a compliant wall is the first requirement. A snug, arterial puncture around a small catheter minimizes pericatheter oozing and hastens haemostasis at the end of the procedure. In our hospital we use 5F catheters which are small but provide adequate torque control. Other centres use even smaller catheters. To facilitate single wall puncture, needles with Doppler attachments may be used.

Once access to the artery has been secured a 5F pigtail catheter is passed into the abdominal aorta. A flush aortic and bilateral study is then obtained to demonstrate the arterial tree from just above the renal arteries to the feet. The puncture site should be observed continuously and digital pressure applied if bleeding occurs.

Setting a clear objective

Once the full diagnostic study has been completed the radiologist and vascular surgeon must agree on the plan. In our experience the best management is usually self-evident when each has experience of the other's techniques and skills. Disputes between the disciplines are very unusual. It is not always easy to identify precisely which lesion is responsible for the ischaemia (Figure 4.7) and it is at this point that the benefits of a clear history, supported by previous investigations, may be invaluable. This consultation should end with the setting of a clear objective: a trial of lysis in a particular artery with re-assessment at an agreed time, never more than 12 hours later.

Crossing the aortic bifurcation

The 5F pigtail catheter is then replaced with a 5F side-winder 1 catheter. This is passed up into the aortic arch where its configuration is formed. The catheter is then brought down the aorta, rotating it to avoid the tip catching on atheromatous plaques or entering side vessels. An alternative to rotating the catheter is to pass a J-shaped guidewire through the tip of the catheter so that 4 or 5 cm are extruded from it and then simply to pull both distally. The distal limb of the catheter is then passed under fluoroscopic control into the common iliac artery. If thrombus is situated in the common iliac artery a side-winder catheter with a longer distal limb, for example a side-winder 2 or 3, may be embedded in the thrombus, and an exchange of catheters need not then be carried out.

If the occlusion is more distal, then a straight catheter or one with a small distal curve will need to be used. In this event a heavy duty J-shaped guidewire should be passed distally as far as possible, preferably into the mid-superficial femoral artery. This is necessary to give adequate anchorage for the passage of the second catheter.

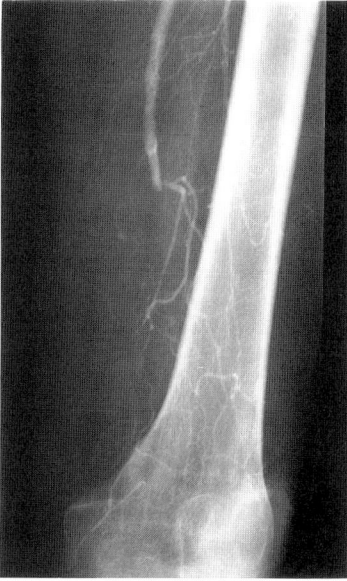

(a)

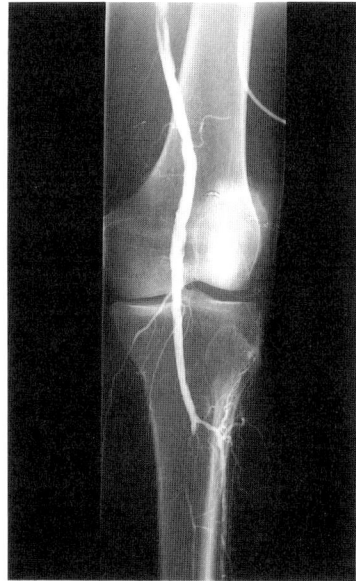

(b)

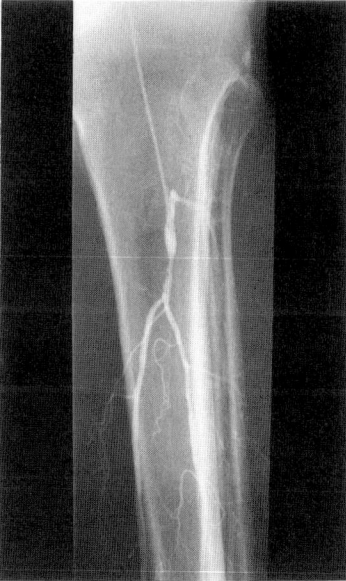

(c)

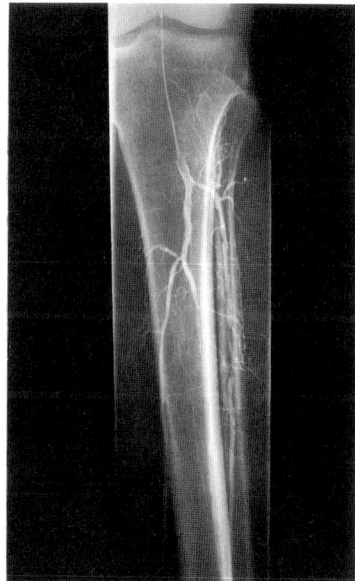

(d)

Figure 4.7 Which lesion is responsible for the ischaemia? (a) A left superficial femoral artery occlusion. (b) Successful thrombolysis of the femoro-popliteal segment with recovery of ankle pulses but occlusion of tibio-peroneal trunk. (c) Continued distal lysis revealed atheromatous stricture of tibio-peroneal trunk. (d) Successful distal angioplasty

Several problems may arise when attempting to pass the second catheter over the guidewire. The catheter may loop into the aorta pulling the guidewire out of the iliac origin. This may be prevented first by passing the guidewire as far as possible into the superficial femoral artery and secondly by the way in which the second catheter is moved over the guidewire at the aortic bifurcation. This should be in a series of short jerking movements rather than a smooth push.

Sometimes the guidewire will pass repeatedly into the internal iliac artery. Often this does not provide adequate anchorage for the passage of the second catheter, particularly if the bifurcation is tortuous. The problem may be overcome in one of two ways. The first method is by pulling the proximal limb of the side-winder inferiorly thereby elevating the distal limb; the J guidewire then bounces over the origin of the internal iliac artery. The second technique is to leave the guidewire in the internal iliac artery and pass a Cobra 1 catheter over the bifurcation. The distal curve of the catheter may then be turned so that it is pointing away from the internal iliac artery. The guidewire can then be passed into the external iliac artery and beyond. Using these techniques catheters can be passed from the groin into the contra-lateral superficial femoral, popliteal or tibial vessels in the majority of cases.

Embedding the catheter

Having passed the catheter to the required level it is then embedded about 2 cm into the obstruction and the thrombolytic infusion commenced. It is essential that the thrombolytic agent accumulates in the thrombus and is not washed away by adjacent blood flow. Normally a catheter with a few side holes 1–2 cm from the tip is chosen. The infusate is prepared by dissolving streptokinase powder in normal saline to give a final concentration of 100 u/ml. This is infused at a rate of 50 ml/h (5000 iu/h). If the thrombus is hard and the catheter cannot be embedded then it may be useful to infuse streptokinase just proximal to the thrombus until it softens and can then be entered. The catheter should then be securely fixed with adhesive tape to prevent movement. No dressing should be used since this would conceal bleeding which is best controlled by digital pressure and local mopping.

The infusion

This should be set up and running before the patient leaves the radiology department. The approximate volume of fluid within the dead space of an angiographic catheter is 1.5 ml. With low infusion rates the catheter will not be filled quickly enough and there will be prolonged periods of fluid stasis, but high rates of infusion risk fluid overload. The line is cleared by first running the pump at 900 ml/h for 30 seconds (7.5 ml). We recommend that infusion rates of 50 ml/h should be used. This compromise gives good flow with a minimal risk of fluid overload, even if continued for more than 24 hours. The infusion should be administered by an accurate volumetric pump. Syringe drivers with a maximum volume of 50 ml are unsuitable for continuous treatment.

Many centres use adjuvant intra-arterial heparin to reduce the risk of pericatheter thrombosis. Some series have reported a high incidence of this complication but in our experience of well over one hundred patients it has not been a serious problem. It is likely that heparin augments the risk of bleeding from streptokinase yet does not increase the lytic potency of the drug and we prefer to rely on brisk pericatheter flow to avoid pericatheter thrombosis.

Nursing care during infusion

A written protocol and experienced nurses are essential for the safe conduct of a thrombolytic infusion. In our hospital the necessary level of skill, supervision and continuity of care is available only on the intensive care unit. In elective cases bowel preparation with suppositories should be given in advance to avoid disturbance during infusion and early urinary catheterization (or the use of slipper bedpans for females) may be helpful. Aseptic technique and close observation of the arterial catheters must be combined with regular clinical records for the early detection of deterioration or haemorrhage.

When the infusion is running satisfactorily the patient should be transferred to the intensive care unit. It is vital that the infusion is not switched off or allowed to stop during transfer. Throughout the patient is nursed flat with only one pillow and kept 'nil by mouth' except for sips of water. Regular observations of pulse, blood pressure, peripheral perfusion and urine output should be carried out and in particular a careful watch kept for any hint of occult bleeding, the first symptom of which may be abdominal pain or hypotension. Treatment is prolonged, uncomfortable and at times painful and there is no reason to withhold adequate analgesia and sedation so that the patient can be as comfortable as possible and is able to lie still. Allergic reactions occur in about 4% of patients[32] and it may be necessary to stop the streptokinase infusion or change to t-PA. Pretreatment with steroids will not always prevent allergic reactions[33]. Fortunately anaphylaxis occurs in fewer than 1%[34]. At agreed intervals, but never more than 12 hours, the patient should have further angiography and forward repositioning of the catheter as lysis progresses distally. This may be done in the radiology department, particularly if angioplasty is likely to be needed, or by a single shot arteriogram carried out on the intensive care unit. For this we use portable equipment and 10–20 ml of non-ionic contrast medium.

Angioplasty

Approximately one-third of our patients required percutaneous transluminal angioplasty. Iliac angioplasty is sometimes used as a preliminary to the passage of an infusion catheter to minimize pericatheter stasis but more distally placed lesions usually require a second ipsi-lateral puncture. In this case it is essential that the contra-lateral catheter is retained and simply perfused with heparinized saline for the rest of the procedure.

The timing of angioplasty may be critical as it is important to re-establish maximal flow as soon as possible (Figure 4.8). Pulsatile flow not only helps to avoid pericatheter thrombosis but also to distribute the thrombolytic agent and to dissolve thrombus. It is therefore important to dilate stenoses

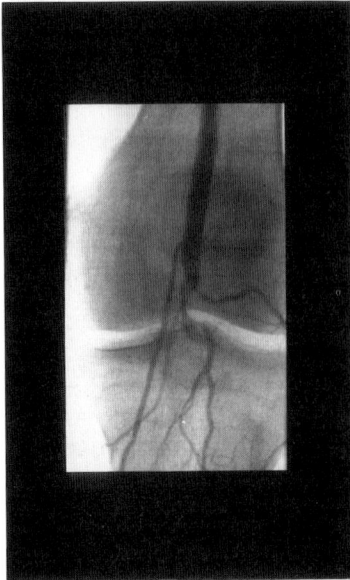

(a)

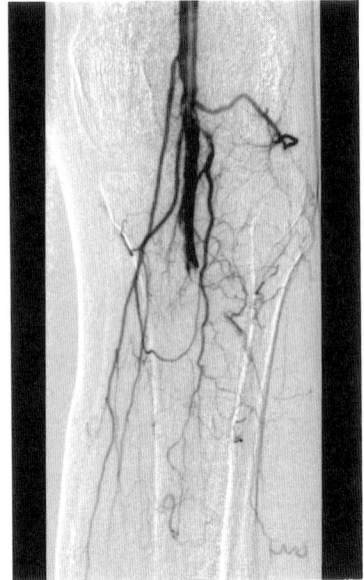

(b)

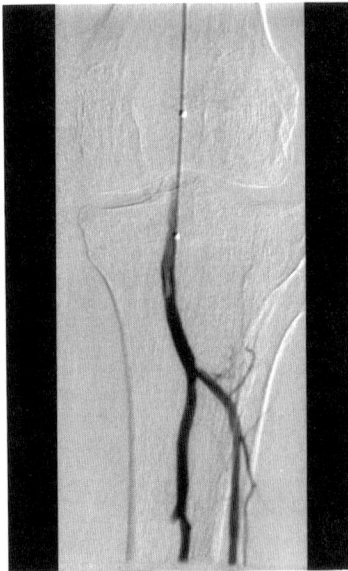

(c)

Figure 4.8 The timing of angioplasty may be critical. (a) Popliteal artery occlusion. (b) During thrombolysis an irregular stricture was demonstrated. (c) Early angioplasty followed by thrombolysis produced a good result

as soon as the obstructing thrombus has been cleared from both the stenotic ring and from the artery just beyond. If the catheter is simply passed through the stenosis and further lytic agent infused, lysis may be slow and pericatheter thrombosis more likely. Angioplasty balloons mounted on shafts which are 5F gauge or less are now available and it is not usually necessary to make a large arterial puncture to carry out angioplasty.

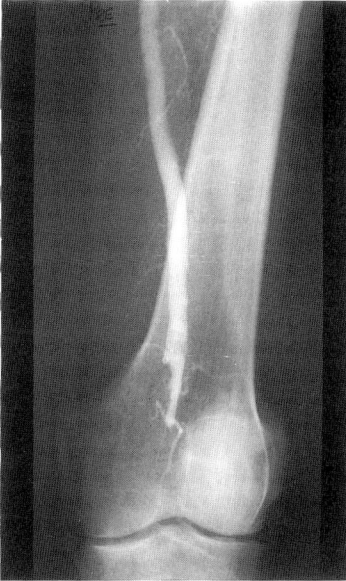

(a)

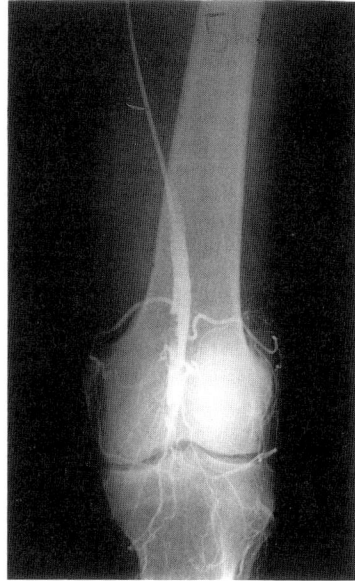

(b)

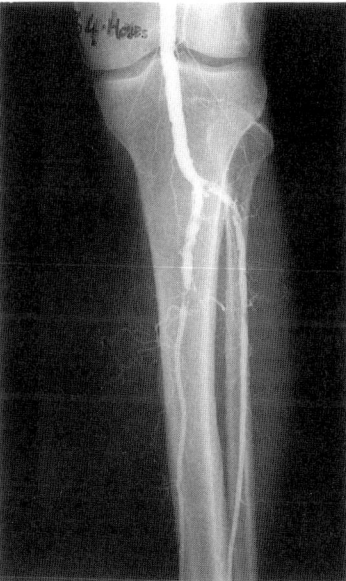

(c)

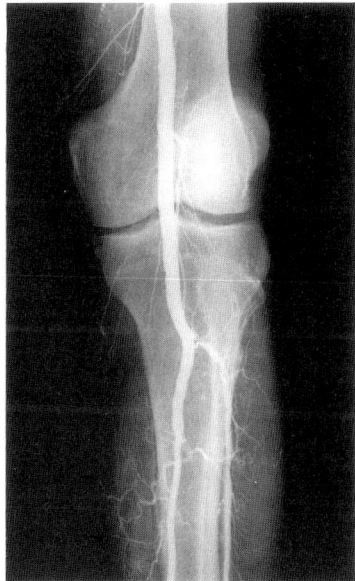

(d)

Figure 4.9 (a) Thrombotic occlusion of popliteal artery. (b) Thrombolysis reveals atheromatous stricture but occluding lesion was actually embolic. (c) Further thrombolysis improved the flow but could not clear the embolic occlusion. (d) Surgical embolectomy was required to restore the foot pulses. A small amount of residual debris in anterior tibial artery could not be cleared

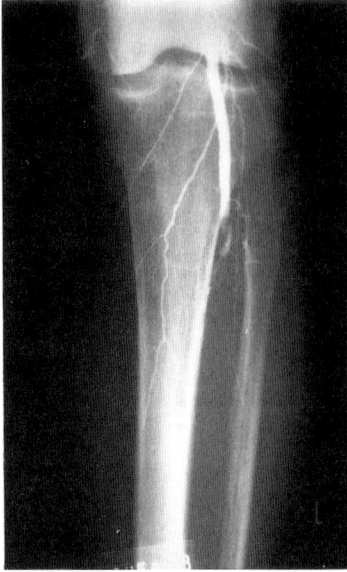 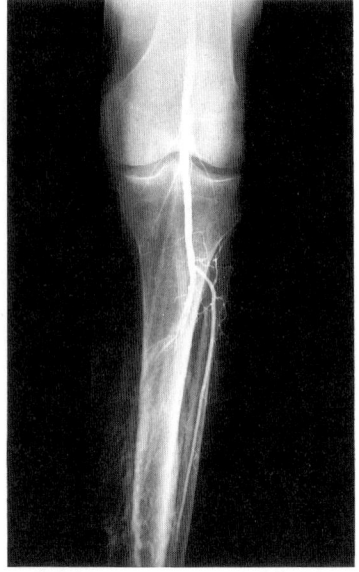

(a)   (b)

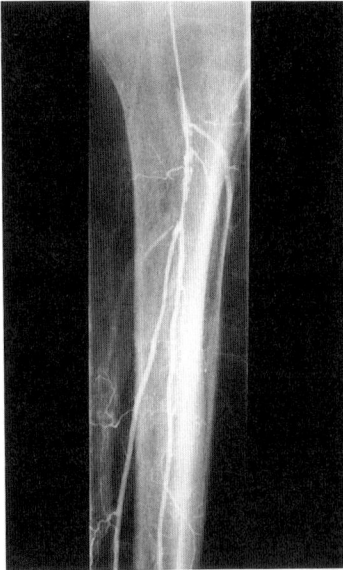 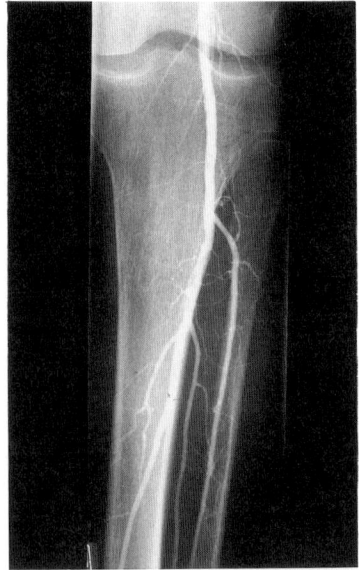

(c)   (d)

Figure 4.10 Combination of lysis and aspiration embolectomy. (a) Embolic occlusion of distal popliteal artery. (b) Anterior tibial artery re-opened with thrombolysis. (c) Aspiration embolectomy of the tibio-peroneal trunk. (d) Combination of aspiration and thrombolysis produced normal distal vessels

The treatment of the cause of the thrombosis is vital if there is to be any hope of long-term benefit. Sometimes this will require angioplasty, sometimes surgical removal of debris (Figure 4.9) and occasionally a bypass operation but in all cases, as vascular surgeons have learned, a satisfactory completion arteriogram must be obtained to confirm the likelihood of sustained patency. Residual defects must be corrected at once. Capillary flow and the return of distal pulses is encouraging but a good result cannot be assumed unless the completion arteriogram is free from significant stenoses, debris or dissection. Return of pedal pulses may occur despite residual obstruction and may be misleadingly optimistic. Arteriographic proof of success is better.

Sometimes only part of the thrombus will be lysed. This is particularly likely after systemic embolism when lysis may dissolve fresh propagation clot but leave the mature cardiac thrombus intact. Again the return of pulses should not be taken to indicate a satisfactory outcome. Re-thrombosis is very likely and clot suction or surgical removal is required for sustained success (Figure 4.10).

When distal vessels are being treated it is useful to administer a vasodilator such as intra-arterial glyceryl trinitrate (GTN) 100–200 μg over 1 minute combined with a GTN patch (5 mg) applied to the skin.

Completion of lysis

When lysis is complete 1000 u heparin should be administered through the catheter. The streptokinase infusion should then be replaced by an intra-arterial infusion of heparin 800–1000 u/h. At a later stage, not less than 4 hours after the streptokinase infusion (2 hours in the case of t-PA), the catheters may be removed, maintaining the patient on intravenous heparin, the dose depending on the result of the APTT. It is probably wise to keep the patient in bed for about 12 hours after treatment. Thrombolysis and heparin may be followed by warfarin or low-dose aspirin (75 mg daily). If longer-term anticoagulation is foreseen at the beginning of treatment, warfarin can be started as thrombolysis begins. The decision whether to maintain the patient on long-term anticoagulation with warfarin or to use a platelet inhibitor such as aspirin will depend upon the anticipated patency of the vessel at the end of the procedure. If there is a good chance of long-term patency with a fast flow in the vessels and minimal stenoses, then the patient will normally be treated adequately by aspirin. In the presence of unrelieved stenoses or multiple untreatable occlusions, long-term warfarin may be preferred although scientific evidence of benefit is not yet available and, particularly in the elderly, long-term warfarin carries an annual 5% risk of serious bleeding[35]. In some patients long-term anticoagulation will be required for coexistent atrial fibrillation or because of synthetic cardiac valves.

Thrombolysis by the bolus technique

An alternative to infusing the thrombolytic agent is the repeated injection of a concentrated bolus of lytic drug into the thrombus. This technique was first published by Hess[8] who injected aliquots of 1000 u streptokinase every 3 minutes, advancing the catheter as lysis progressed. His technique was introduced before the safety of low dose infusion was established and the advantage of the technique was that less streptokinase was administered and the procedure was terminated as soon as lysis had been achieved. Bolus injections of 5 mg t-PA every 15 minutes is an alternative method[36]. The main disadvantage is that the operator has to be present with the patient in the radiological department for relatively long periods to give every injection and in a busy district general hospital where there is intense demand on limited equipment and the radiologist's time, infusion may be preferred. Rapid lysis by the repeated bolus technique extends the repertoire of thrombolysis into the treatment of severe ischaemia, even perhaps the acute white leg, but there is little firm evidence to suggest that this technique is better than urgent surgery (see Chapter 5).

Distal embolization

It is not uncommon for distal embolization of thrombus to occur during thrombolytic therapy and this may be quite alarming (Figure 4.11). Often the foot, which previously appeared viable, becomes white and mottled and the patient may experience considerable pain. Usually these embolic thrombi are small and are a complication of successful therapy. The patient should be treated with analgesia and further sedation if necessary and the thrombolytic infusion continued. This will usually result in clearance of the embolic material.

Resistant clot in small vessels

Following lysis of most of the thrombus after embolization a small amount of resistant clot is sometimes encountered. This usually represents a nidus of old, organized intracardiac thrombus. It is usually small in volume and can only be removed by surgery or by percutaneous aspiration.

In other cases, particularly after angioplasty, it may be difficult to embed the 5F catheter into thrombus below the knee. The procedure of choice is then to advance a guidewire containing an injection lumen coaxially through the infusion catheter into the thrombus. A Touhy–Borst adaptor should be used and thrombolytic solution infused into both catheters (Figure 4.12). Lysis by the bolus technique may be preferred at this point to achieve rapid results under direct vision using either streptokinase or t-PA every 15 minutes.

Retrograde lysis

In some hospitals it is usual to pass the catheter under fluoroscopic control through the thrombus to its distal end and gradually withdraw it as lysis progresses. This technique may reduce the risk of distal embolization. A disadvantage of this technique may be the lack of pulsatile flow which should aid local mixing and lysis, but an advantage is that as lysis proceeds the catheter may be pulled back into further thrombus simply by measuring the length on a single X-ray film. Further visits to the radiology department for forward repositioning may thus be avoided.

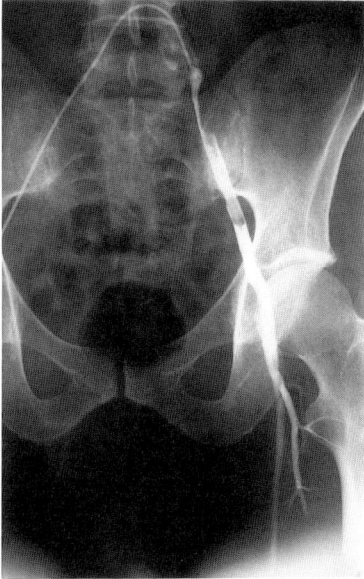

(a)

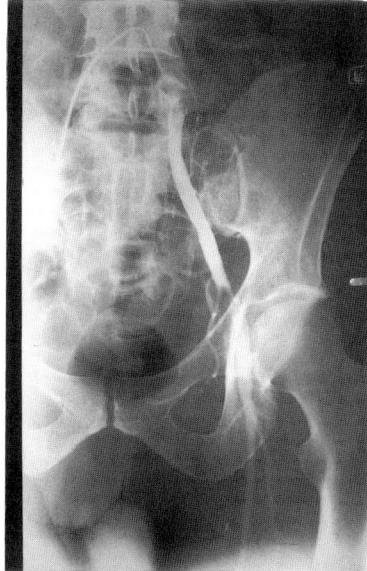

(b)

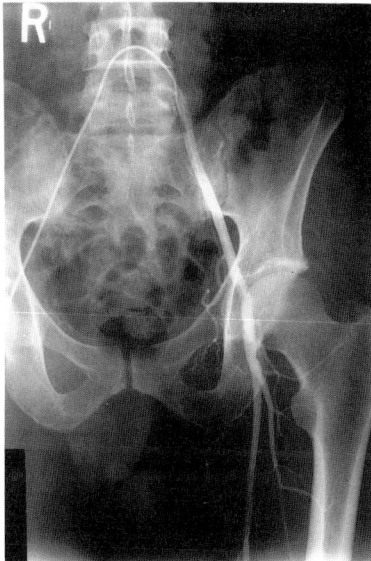

(c)

Figure 4.11 Distal embolization during
thrombolysis. (a) Thrombotic occlusion of
left common iliac artery due to underlying
atheroma. (b) Clot migrated distally during
thrombolysis. (c) Continued thrombolysis
restored the circulation

Brachial puncture

High brachial puncture may be used for the insertion of thrombolysis
catheters when thrombus occurs in the abdominal aorta, mesenteric or renal
arteries or where the approach from the contra-lateral groin is precluded.
The disadvantage of this approach is that if bleeding occurs within the tight

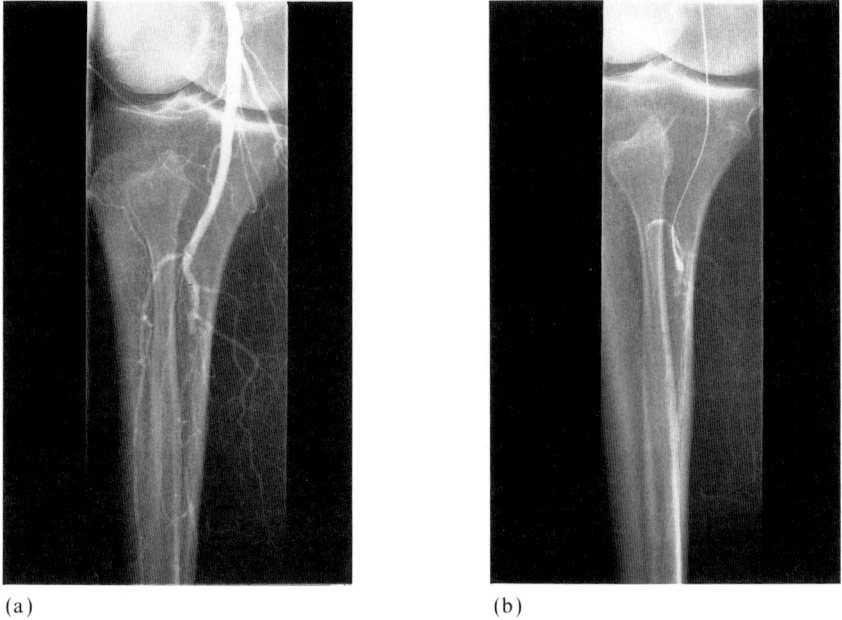

(a)   (b)

Figure 4.12 Thrombolysis of distal embolization. (a) After successful thrombolysis of right superficial femoral artery occlusion, there was distal embolization to the calf vessels. (b) A lumenal guidewire positioned for distal thrombolysis

compartment of the neurovascular fascial sheath there is a significant risk of neurological damage. Both here and in the groin where the femoral nerve is vulnerable, tense haematoma must never be neglected. Surgical decompression by haematoma evacuation and direct repair of the arterial puncture is required to prevent permanent neurological damage. Axillary artery puncture should be avoided as compression of the axillary artery following removal of the lysis catheter can be more difficult than compression of the brachial artery in the upper arm. Low brachial puncture in the antecubital fossa may be used but the greater length of catheter required is a disadvantage and reduces torque control. The possibility of pericatheter thrombosis and damage both to the arterial wall and to the median and ulnar nerves is greater when a low brachial puncture is used.

Thrombolysis in grafts

Thrombosis in grafts is an increasing problem. When it occurs within a month of implantation it is usually the result in an error in selection or a technical defect. The selection of a patient with inadequate inflow or outflow means the reconstruction is doomed to failure even if technically perfect: if there is a technical defect in the graft itself or at the anastomosis, early thrombosis will be likely. Thrombolysis of propagated clot may then help to show the cause but its use should be limited because of the risk of bleeding from suture lines within 1 month of initial surgery. Intra-operative thrombolysis during surgical re-exploration of a thrombosed graft in the early post-operative period may be safer since it can be given into the arrested circulation of a limb with much greater control than is the case with a prolonged infusion[37].

Occlusion more than 1 month after implantation is often the result of a progressive stenosis. A regular programme of graft surveillance may help to prevent a developing stenosis from progressing to complete occlusion[38]. It is certain that revision before thrombosis has a much better chance of long-term benefit than treatment of an established occlusion, particularly in autogenous vein grafts. These are prone to develop stenoses in the body of the graft and suffer permanent intimal damage when thrombosis occurs. Stenoses are much better treated by early surgery, either enlarging the stricture with a vein patch or providing flow around it by local bypass or jump grafting. Both vein and synthetic grafts may develop anastomotic strictures, usually involving the whole circumference of the anastomosis, due to neointimal hyperplasia. Anti-platelet drugs may reduce the development of neointimal hyperplasia and should always be used[39] unless there is a specific contra-indication. Some strictures may develop because of fibrosis and contracture in the deeper layers of the anastomosis resulting in a concentric fibrous stricture. Prophylactic measures are again to be preferred since the completed thrombosis poses difficulties in catheterization of the graft. Balloon angioplasty is less effective in permanently dilating fibrous strictures than in dilating atheromatous lesions of the native arteries. Neointimal hyperplasia may also affect large-bore synthetic grafts, progressively narrowing the whole length of the graft. This is best treated by removal using thrombo-embolectomy or endarterectomy techniques. Though recommended by some authors[40], we do not now use thrombolysis to re-open a retroperitoneally implanted Dacron graft since occult and dangerous bleeding may occur even years after implantation. Extravasation through the wall of a subcutaneously implanted Dacron or polytetrafluoroethelyne (PTFE) graft may also occur but this is usually obvious and more easily controlled. Infra-inguinal grafts and extra-anatomic reconstructions are therefore particularly suitable for thrombolysis. Obviously, synthetic grafts are not vulnerable to intimal damage but may thrombose without any permanent underlying defect, perhaps because of temporary dehydration, low cardiac output or graft compression. Thrombolysis and anticoagulation may offer a renewed prospect of long-term patency.

Two techniques are available for the dissolution of thrombus within such grafts, the contra-lateral approach, which is the method of first choice, and direct puncture of the graft. Strict asepsis and prophylactic antibiotics are mandatory. Methods of accessing grafts and thrombolytic techniques are discussed in Chapter 6.

Lysis in synthetic grafts may yield curious and unexpected phenomena. Grafts previously impervious to lytic drugs may become very porous when treated for a second time and anastomoses may also leak months or years after implantation, producing false aneurysms. Failed lysis in a synthetic graft may occasionally save the limb by reopening the long thrombosed native artery occlusion for which the graft was done. These bizarre phenomena should remind us that our understanding of the whole process remains incomplete and should encourage a cautious approach.

Popliteal aneurysm

The true prevalence of popliteal aneurysms is unknown but symptoms or complications lead to its discovery in one or two patients in our practice covering 200 000 people each year. Almost all are atherosclerotic although popliteal artery entrapment syndrome, collagen disorders, infection and blunt or penetrating trauma may also cause aneurysms. The condition is said to account for 1 in 5000 hospital admissions and about one popliteal aneurysm presents for every 15 abdominal aortic aneurysms. Many patients harbour small uncomplicated aneurysms for years but a small proportion will present acutely with a limb-threatening thrombosis[41].

The results of surgery for this catastrophe are often poor and are crucially dependent upon the patency of tibial vessels. These may have been blocked by two quite separate processes which, though difficult to distinguish in every patient, have different effects and a different prognosis. The first is distal occlusion due to microembolization of flow thrombus or atheromatous debris from the aneurysm. The acute syndrome resembles postoperative 'trash foot': multiple occlusions of the small vessels of the calf and foot with patchy but severe ischaemia sometimes in the presence of a strong pedal pulse. Minor episodes may go unnoticed leading to slowly progressive but severe ischaemia. The second process is that of tibial vessel atherosclerosis. The distal ischaemia is more generalized and to an extent the small vessels of the foot are protected from distal emboli. These two important mechanisms may co-exist but an attempt must be made to distinguish them clinically and by careful arteriography. Thrombolysis may succeed in reopening the lumen of a recently occluded popliteal aneurysm when that occlusion is due to propagation clot but it is unlikely to improve tibial atherosclerosis or trash foot.

Even in symptomatic limbs the diagnosis of popliteal aneurysm may be missed, although over 90% of symptomatic aneurysms are readily palpable[42] and the increasing use of thrombolysis for acute lower limb ischaemia has led to the identification of popliteal aneurysm as the cause of thrombosis in an increasing number of patients[43].

The best elective treatment for a patent, symptomatic aneurysm is surgical bypass using autogenous vein. When the distal vessels are patent, long-term results are excellent. Some patients have small, uncomplicated and asymptomatic aneurysms which are smooth walled, contain little thrombus and are probably at low risk of complications. These may be managed conservatively particularly where safe thrombolysis is available to offset the low risk of thrombosis[44]. However, this remains controversial. Large symptomatic aneurysms, often associated with generalized arterial ectasia, intralumenal thrombus, distortion of the outflow tract, atherosclerotic or embolic distal occlusions and obstruction of the popliteal vein, are quite a different problem and when they present acutely with severe ischaemia there is a risk that the most intensive management will not save the limb[45]. Surgery alone will succeed only if the run-off is clear. Pre-operative or intra-operative thrombolysis improves the outflow in the majority of cases of acute thrombosis and may be required occasionally when a further aneurysm complicates a previously successful aneurysm bypass.

Some patients will not respond to thrombolysis because there is resistant debris in the small vessels of the foot; neither are they likely to benefit from surgical thrombectomy and bypass. Some are more fortunate because the distal occlusions are due to atherosclerosis of the calf vessels and careful arteriography and Doppler studies will reveal patent vessels at or below the ankle to which a successful bypass may be made. Lysis of propagation clot may aid the demonstration of this potential.

Where time allows we recommend a trial of lysis by infusion, hoping to prepare the patient for a successful bypass (or long-term anticoagulation if they are unfit for surgery). The catheter tip should be positioned within or beyond the aneurysm, the aim being to re-open occluded distal vessels to enable successful bypass. When time is short, surgical exploration with thrombectomy, intra-operative thrombolysis and arteriography are required to prepare for bypass grafting and these constitute the preferred management. The outflow remains the key to success. Even a patent graft may not save the foot if distal vessels remain acutely obstructed.

Thrombolysis in arteriovenous shunts

Thrombosis in synthetic conduits may occur because flow is reduced by compression or angulation and the injection of a bolus of streptokinase or t-PA will usually clear fresh propagation clot. Quick action will often preserve a valuable shunt, which may be needed for long-term therapy. Prolonged stasis will however cause intimal damage on either side of the shunt and recurrent thrombosis even if the flow disorder is corrected. This will require a new shunt at a new site, as will any evidence of infection.

Local treatment of shunts is possible using 10 000–25 000 u of strepto-kinase in the thrombosed shunt. This is sealed on the venous side by forceps. A syringe is attached to the arterial side to form an air cushion against which the artery can pulsate. The treatment may be repeated after 30–45 minutes. Alternatively, 5 mg of t-PA may be used.

Thrombolysis in intravenous catheters

Ideally this should never be necessary since proper management of central venous lines includes the maintenance of continuous forward flow. When retrograde flow has occurred, thrombus in the lumen should not simply be extruded into the circulation by syringe pressure but should be lysed by a small volume of injected streptokinase or t-PA. It is essential to check that the catheter is satisfactorily positioned in the lumen of a great vein and not, for example, passing up a jugular vein or down the opposite arm. Asepsis must be maintained. Thrombosis in intravenous catheters secondary to infection or thrombophlebitis in the vein should not be treated by thrombolysis. These are highly dangerous conditions with a risk of septicaemia or major venous thrombosis, and immediate removal of the catheter and culture of its tip are vital.

Intra-arterial thrombolysis for massive venous thrombosis (phlegmasia cerulea dolens)

A recent report of this application of intra-arterial thrombolysis with surgical thrombectomy[46] suggests that it may be of value where massive venous obstruction occludes arterial inflow. Results of further experiences are awaited with interest.

Thrombolysis after intra-arterial injection

Thrombolytic drugs, heparin, prostaglandins and vasodilators have been used to treat the effects of accidental and deliberate intra-arterial injection of toxic chemicals. While useful in removing propagation clot, the outcome depends on the degree of spasm and endothelial damage. Unfortunately the use of 'home-made' drugs (often oral preparations mixed in water) frequently causes irreversible endothelial damage and transmural necrosis.

Dealing with the cause

Thrombolysis does not stand alone. This recent technique should always be seen in relation to the three causes of thrombosis enunciated by Virchow in the mid 1800s, when he categorized the aetiology of thrombosis into factors related to stasis, abnormality of the vessel wall and coagulability of the blood. In a small number of our cases no anatomical abnormality was found and there was no explanation of the thrombosis. Our efforts were then directed towards reducing the thrombotic potential of the blood, for example by treating polycythaemia or by giving anticoagulation with warfarin. Improving cardiac output and increasing mobility may also help to prevent recurrence but the best opportunities for long-term success occur when a stenosis is corrected by angioplasty or surgery (Figure 4.13).

Unless the cause of the thrombosis is identified and rectified, re-thrombosis will almost always occur. To subject the patient to an uncomfortable and invasive procedure only to suffer a relapse in a few weeks or months is to have done the patient a major disservice. In some cases the thrombolytic infusion may demonstrate that the situation is hopeless; for example a patient with no run-off. Further therapy is fruitless. Although disappointing, this is useful information because ineffective treatment can be avoided and amputation advised. In other cases thrombolytic infusion may demonstrate one or more stenoses as the cause of the thrombosis. These should be dealt with by angioplasty and it may be necessary to perform angioplasty of the tibial vessels as well as of the larger arteries.

In the case of grafts, stenoses may be due to intimal hyperplasia or scarring around the anastomosis and these are easily recognized. In some cases thrombosis is caused by kinking of the graft, particularly when the knee is flexed, and this abnormality is not so easily detected. Full assessment needs to include demonstration of the graft both in the neutral position to show any twist or kink and with flexion of any joint which is crossed.

Haematological monitoring during thrombolysis

This is frequently advised and baseline observations of bleeding and clotting measurements including fibrinogen, APTT, blood count and platelets are

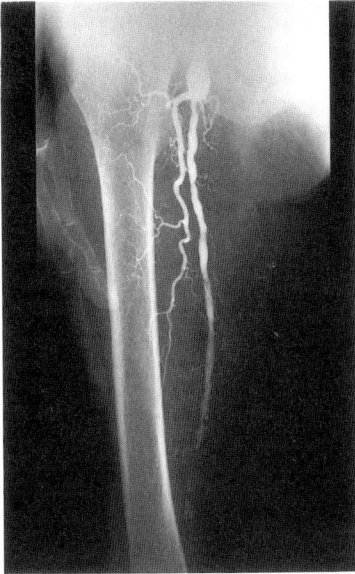

(a)

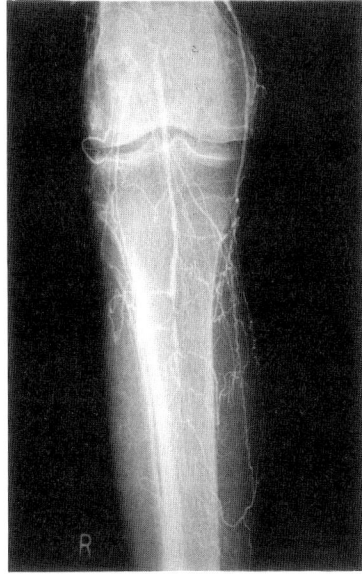

(b)

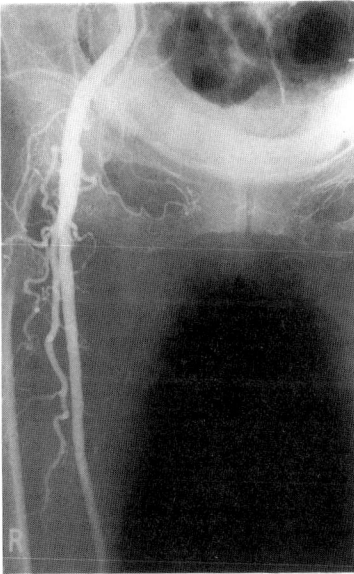

(c)

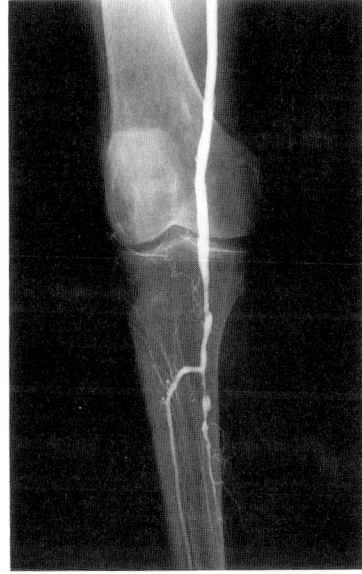

(d)

Figure 4.13 (a) Occluded right femoro-popliteal graft. (b) Run off below occluded graft showed patent but diseased tibial vessels. (c) Graft patency restored by thrombolysis. (d) Outflow restricted by atheromatous disease in the native popliteal and tibial arteries which requires angioplasty for prolonged graft patency

usual. Measurement of fibrin degradation products (e.g. D-dimer) should be done if disseminated intravascular coagulation is suspected. Existing anti-coagulation with warfarin should be reversed to the low therapeutic range and repeated measurements of these parameters should be carried out every 12–24 hours. If fibrinogen levels fall below 1 g/l (normal range 2–4 g/l) or the thrombin time ratio rises above 1.5 (normal range 1.00–1.15) the rate of infusion should be halved. If fibrinogen drops below 0.5 g/l, the infusion should be suspended. Unfortunately changes in haematological measure-ments have not proved to be a reliable indicator of the risk of major bleeding but it is unwise to ignore the evidence when the results suggest deterioration.

The treatment of haemorrhage

Haemorrhage amounting to more than a little seepage around the arterial catheter is a sign that the infusion should be stopped. The half-lives of both streptokinase (23 minutes) and t-PA (8 minutes) are sufficiently short that bleeding due to thrombolysis itself should stop within the hour and the catheters should be left in place until then. Continued ooze can be treated by tranexamic acid (Cyklokapron) but there is a risk of arterial thrombosis. If the patient is severely defibrinogenated, fresh frozen plasma or 8–10 units of cryoprecipitate may be used. Aprotinin (Trasylol), which has been found useful to reduce bleeding in surgical operations when the patient is heparinized such as cardiac bypass[47], has yet to be evaluated in thrombolysis. More profuse or continued bleeding suggests an arterial (or occasionally venous) laceration. Direct digital pressure, compressing but not occluding the vessel, may succeed but continued bleeding requires surgical repair. It is important to appreciate that the arterial puncture may be several centimetres away from the skin puncture and precise point pressure on the defect is required. Localization may be aided by ultrasound imaging[48]. Surgical repair of arterial punctures is occasionally required when bleeding continues despite correction of the coagulopathy and effective local pressure[49].

The most serious risk of thrombolysis is stroke and any suspicion of such an accident should lead to immediate suspension of the infusion and an urgent computed tomography or magnetic resonance scan. Confirmed haemorrhage rules out further thrombolysis.

Surgical intervention

This is required to repair vessel damage, to remove resistant thrombus and atheromatous debris and to carry out surgical angioplasty or bypass. Conventional vascular surgical techniques are used with systemic hepariniz-ation, minimal dissection and an atraumatic technique of vessel control and exploration. Arteriotomies in normal vessels should be transverse and repaired with fine interrupted prolene sutures. In atheromatous vessels or where an anastomosis may be required a vertical arteriotomy is needed. This can be closed by a vein patch without risk of stenosis. Operative arteriography to confirm a satisfactory result is mandatory.

Occasionally patients who have undergone thrombolysis and angioplasty present with the late development of a false aneurysm at the site of the arterial puncture[50]. Most remain small and resolve spontaneously but, if

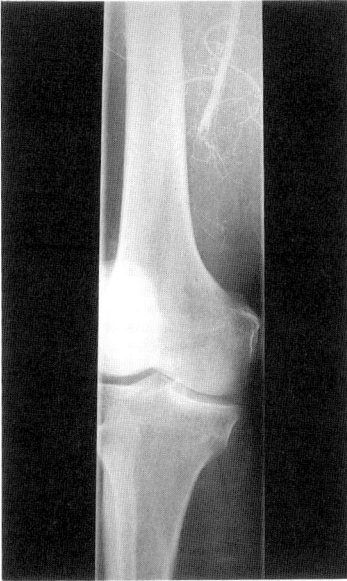

(a)

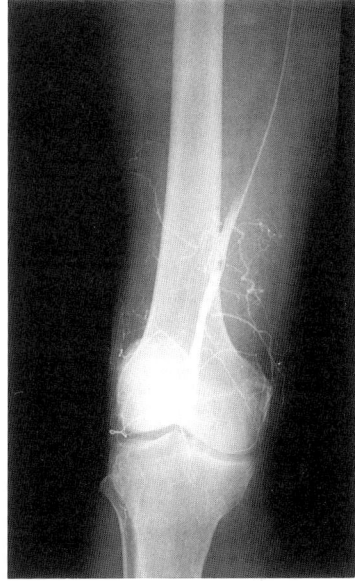

(b)

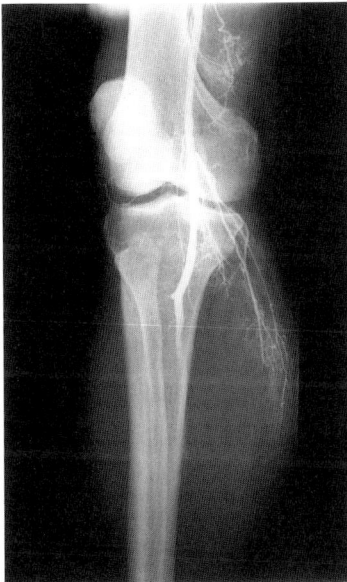

(c)

Figure 4.14 Successful thrombolysis but poor clinical outcome. (a) The viability of the limb was initially in doubt but angiography revealed a distal superficial femoral artery occlusion. (b) Thrombolysis removed propagated thrombus. (c) Thrombolysis reopened vessels down to the calf but severe compartment compression syndrome was shown by tapering and occlusion of deep arteries and tufting of vessels in calf. Circulation was improved and the limb retained, but function was poor due to ischaemic muscle fibrosis

ultrasound imaging confirms the aneurysm to have a narrow neck and to be expanding, direct surgical repair is required. Ultrasound location may be followed by occlusion with precise pressure using the ultrasound probe[51]. If surgery is required formal mobilization of the vessel is usually unnecessary unless there has been delay, or infection is making the arterial defect larger.

When it is small, firm external compression will allow incision of the aneurysm and direct suture. By contrast, full exposure is a major procedure.

Acute limb deterioration during thrombolysis

There have been several reports of progressive and refractory thrombosis during thrombolytic infusion. The condition must be distinguished from early rethrombosis after successful lysis which is a well-described complication which may occur days or months after successful treatment. In severe cases of acute limb deterioration irreversible ischaemia develops during the infusion despite initial lysis[52]. The rapid development and intractability of this phenomenon suggests massive distal embolization with or without coagulopathy, reperfusion syndrome or compartment compression (Figure 4.14). The exact incidence is unknown but it is probably less than 3% overall, although up to 13% in the treatment of popliteal aneurysm[53]. Amputation rates are high and urgent surgery is recommended.

Care after thrombolysis

Crossover heparin, aspirin and warfarin

There is controversy over whether or not to give heparin with thrombolytic drugs. There is no evidence to suggest that it enhances the process of thrombolysis and it may even retard it. We do not use concurrent heparin because we are concerned not to increase the risk of bleeding. Heparin certainly does not confer any benefit during thrombolysis with t-PA[54]. Evidence that it causes bleeding during arterial thrombolysis is anecdotal but in the treatment of venous thrombosis low-dose streptokinase 10 000 u/h and low-dose heparin 417 u/h were shown to be associated with more deaths, haemorrhages and strokes than high dose 100 000 u/h streptokinase[55]. It is however essential to use heparin after thrombolysis, particularly to cover further procedures such as angioplasty or surgery or while awaiting the delayed action of warfarin. We recommend use of an intra-arterial bolus of 1000 u followed by 800 u/h by intra-arterial infusion. The effect should be monitored by the APTT and the dose adjusted to maintain a satisfactory level, usually an APTT ratio of 1.5–2.5.

All patients should receive long-term therapy with low-dose aspirin unless specifically contra-indicated so that the risk of platelet aggregation in areas of intimal damage or in synthetic grafts is minimized. There is good evidence that aspirin also helps to prevent other cardiovascular complications such as myocardial infarction and stroke in this vulnerable group[56]. Some patients with prosthetic valves or grafts, atrial fibrillation or previous deep vein thrombosis will require long-term warfarin, as may those with a specific risk of thrombosis.

Removing the catheter

Catheters can be removed immediately on completion of thrombolysis but it is generally convenient to allow 2–4 hours for any systemic effects to decline and for the initial infusion of heparin. On withdrawal, continuous firm pressure over the arterial puncture (not the skin puncture) is applied for 15 minutes, while the distal pulse is monitored to make sure that flow is not interrupted. Exact positioning of the pressure is more important than force, particularly in the obese, but control may be made difficult or impossible if a large, tense haematoma has been allowed to develop. Surgical evacuation and direct repair is then to be preferred since persistent tense haematoma encourages both further bleeding and venous compression with the risk of deep vein thrombosis. Nerve compression may also occur leading to protracted weakness. In rare cases troublesome secondary sepsis may follow haematoma formation.

Documenting the result

The physical signs such as colour, pulses and pedal artery pressures which correlate with the final radiographic assessment must be recorded so that deterioration or improvement can be detected. This is particularly important if surgery or angioplasty is planned.

Follow-up

This is required to assess the result and to prevent recurrence. Attendance at a vascular clinic for clinical review should be supported by objective measurements of the result in the vascular laboratory. Ankle pressures may continue to improve for some months after thrombolysis, angioplasty and reconstruction, and stable pressures do not always mean that the treated vessel has remained patent. Ideally follow-up should be by arteriography. Deterioration certainly requires further investigation by duplex ultrasound or angiography. As with vascular grafts a suitable schedule is to review the patient at 1 month and then 3 monthly for a year. Longer intervals are then sufficient, provided that the patient knows he must report any sudden change without delay.

The results of thrombolysis

Assessment of the results

The variation between patients and the uncertain correlation between the fate of the treated vessels and the physical signs makes this a difficult task unless every follow-up assessment includes ultrasound imaging or arteriographic proof of patency. This is practical only in a research setting. Clinical review with Doppler evidence of flow and pressure is sufficient to detect changes important to the patient but may overestimate the technical achievements. Stenoses may recur slowly and new occlusions may develop without worsening symptoms. Other medical problems may impair the patient's mobility and conceal arterial deterioration. Surrogate indicators of patency such as ankle pressures should not be relied upon to justify a procedure although they do help to monitor the progress of an individual.

Results should be expressed as simply as possible and in a way which fits the clinical problem. An assessment of clinical benefit, which is clearly important from the patient's viewpoint, must be supported by unambiguous end-points such as death and amputation. We must always seek scientific proof of the effect of treatment before claiming credit, despite the difficulties in obtaining unequivocal data. Mortality rates in thrombolysis are not greatly influenced by the treatment itself and are therefore useful as indicators of the frailty of the selected population, and particularly useful for making comparisons between series. Mortality rates of 15% within the first month after presentation are common in elderly patients with severe critical ischaemia, as are amputation rates of 20%. Thereafter mortality rates remain high, 40% of patients are dead by 5 years, although the rate of limb loss in survivors is only 10%. The group remains vulnerable both to other fatal cardiovascular complications and the increased rates of malignancy which are found in the elderly. By contrast, patients presenting with intermittent claudication suffer a very low mortality within 1 month of presentation rising to 30% at 5 years. Limb loss is also much less common.

The high rate of attrition in critical ischaemia complicates analysis, as does the fact that mortality may be due to causes other than peripheral vascular disease and that mortality is not greatly influenced by treatment. Analysis of results by the life-table method is therefore inappropriate. Although a widely used and convenient method by which patients can be recruited to a study at any time, the evidence is flawed by concealing the effect of mortality on the group and presenting an oversimplified and falsely optimistic impression of the effects of treatment. It is of limited value, for example, to know that 70% of grafts are patent at 5 years when, due to other effects, only a minority of the patients survive. We have therefore chosen to report our results simply in terms of effective lysis, clinical benefit, death and amputation.

Results of the Guildford protocol

Our initial experience of intra-arterial thrombolysis using streptokinase over 2 years in 26 patients (27 infusions) was reported in 1985[9]. Included in this series were two patients who had thrombolysis for the occluded limb of an intra-abdominal Dacron graft. Lysis in one of these grafts, implanted 5 weeks previously, led to significant retroperitoneal bleeding requiring resuscitation and the transfusion of 6 units of blood. This was associated with a significant drop in fibrinogen over a 16-hour period, although the dose of streptokinase was only 7000 units per hour. This complication which is well recorded by others even late after graft implantation has led us to use a surgical clearance for retroperitoneally implanted synthetic graft occlusion rather than thrombolysis. We also treated a patient with upper limb thrombosis without success and have not pursued this technique due to the intrinsic technical difficulties mentioned above and the theoretical risk of cerebral embolism.

We were however impressed with the power of the technique to reveal unsuspected pathology, particularly in two instances of primary popliteal aneurysms, and in a further instance where a second, recently thrombosed, popliteal aneurysm had developed above a previous graft. This had been carried out for primary popliteal aneurysm 7 years before. Thrombolysis was shown to be effective but not always clinically useful; for example a thrombosed femoro-popliteal graft was re-opened but a stenosis at the origin of the graft and an occluded run-off made long-term success unlikely.

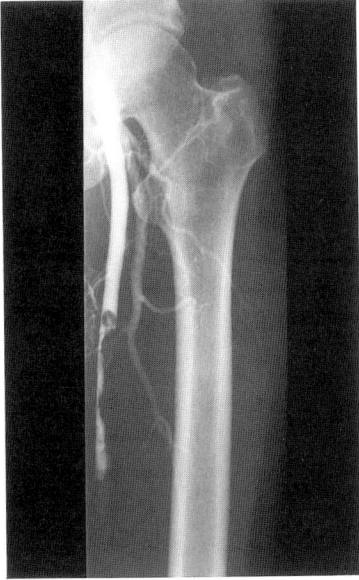

(a)

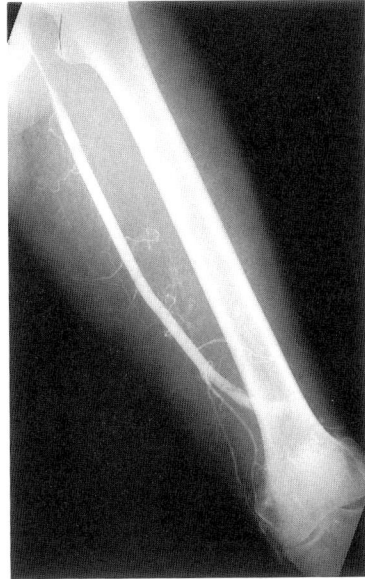

(b)

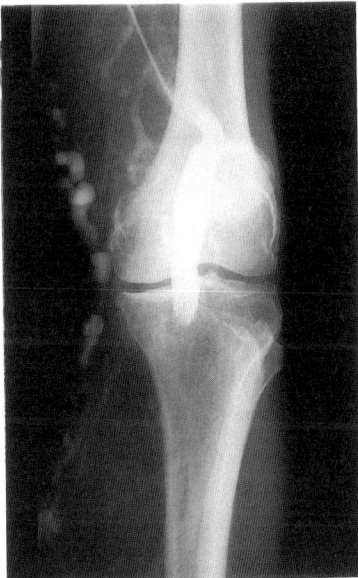

(c)

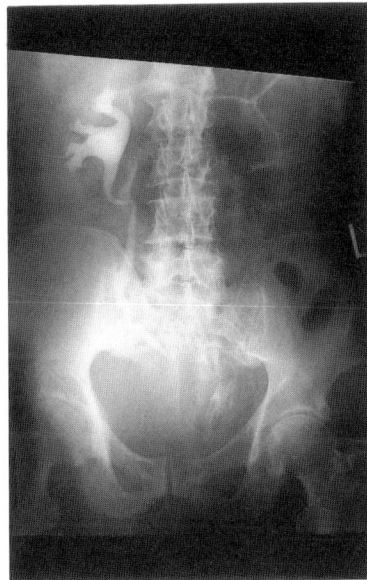

(d)

Figure 4.15 Fatal outcome after retroperitoneal haemorrhage during thrombolysis. (a) Left superficial femoral artery occlusion. (b) Successful thrombolysis in the superficial femoral artery. (c) Continued thrombolysis revealed an unsuspected popliteal aneurysm.
(d) Thrombolysis was discontinued because of retroperitoneal haemorrhage here demonstrated by displacement of the right ureter and bladder to the left. The patient developed aspiration pneumonia during hypovolaemic collapse and died

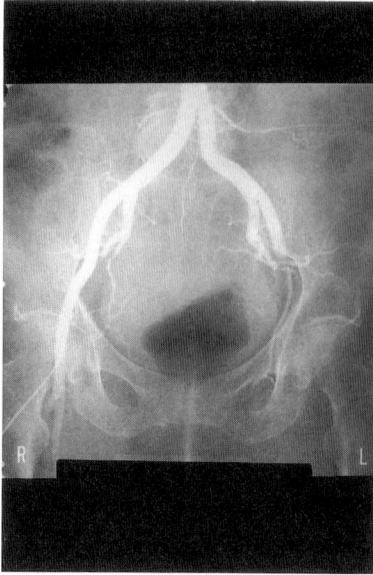

(a)

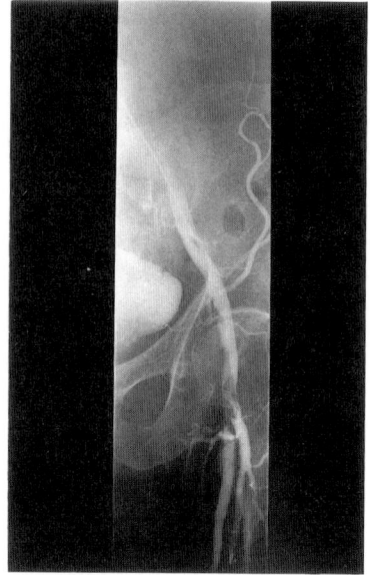

(b)

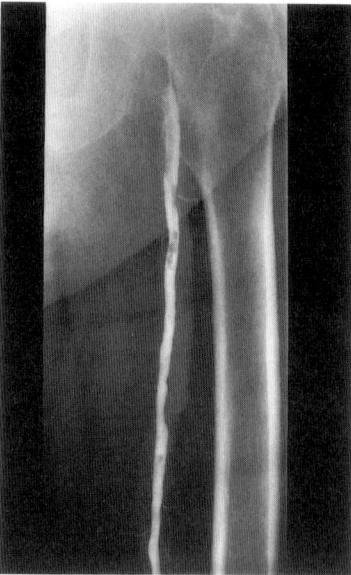

(c)

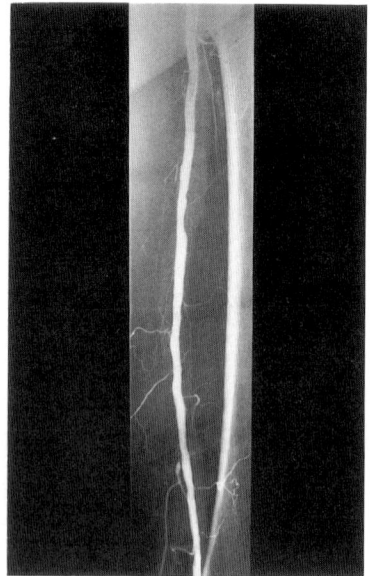

(d)

Figure 4.16 A triumph for perseverance in acute global ischaemia of the left leg; treatment may take several days. (a) Complete occlusion of the left common iliac artery, no distal vessels visualized. (b) Lysis of the common iliac and external iliac arteries. (c), (d) Continued lysis in the common femoral and superficial femoral arteries. (e) Lysis as far as the popliteal artery. (f) Anterior tibial artery origin is re-opened. (g) Further lysis re-opening the anterior tibial artery. (h) No further improvement at the end of this period. The procedure was successfully concluded and the limb saved

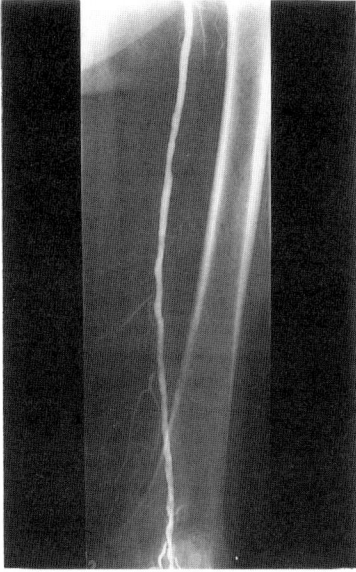

(e)

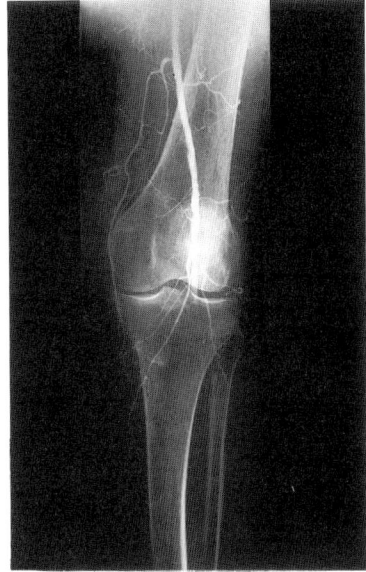

(f)

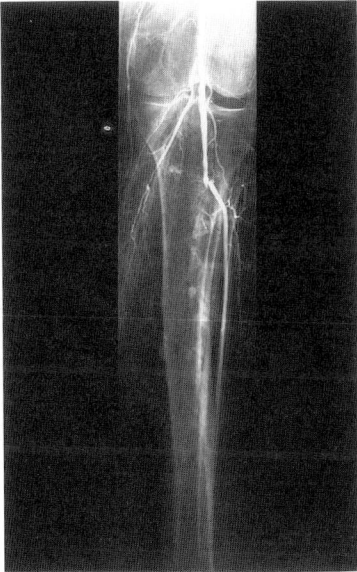

(g)

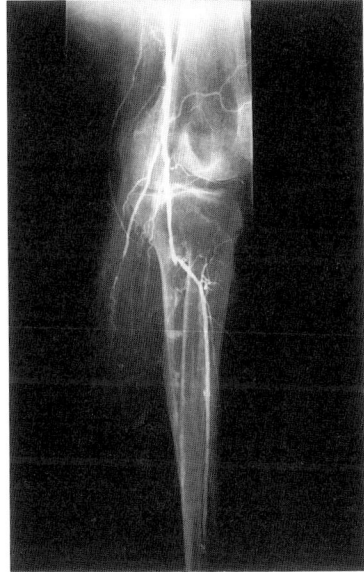

(h)

There was one fatality in the early series due to an intra-abdominal haemorrhage probably caused by the accidental puncture of the external iliac vein (Figure 4.15). Despite successful treatment of the haemorrhage by suture and reversal of the streptokinase with tranexamic acid, the patient died following aspiration of vomit during haemorrhagic shock. Another patient suffered haemorrhage into the popliteal fossa due to continued thrombolytic therapy despite the demonstration of a small false aneurysm at an anastomosis. One patient developed a significant allergy requiring the infusion to be discontinued and two patients showed evidence of distal embolization.

As a result of this experience the selection of patients was modified to exclude those with upper limb thrombosis, and those with retroperitoneally implanted Dacron grafts. Concurrent heparin was no longer used and the dose of streptokinase limited to 5000 or 6000 u/h. We also resolved that, if no improvement was detected after 12 hours of infusion, the treatment should be discontinued and that every effort should be made to correct all arterial defects as soon as possible.

The details of this revised Guildford protocol were published in 1988[10] together with the results from the treatment of 70 patients (72 infusions). Effective lysis was achieved in 52 (72%) of these patients with an average infusion time of 25 hours. A total of 23 (32%) also underwent percutaneous transluminal angioplasty and 19 (26%) required surgery to deal with persistent stenoses, organized thrombus or atheromatous debris. Complications due to bleeding were significantly reduced (to 6%) and the amputation rate to 18%. With increasing experience and more appropriate selection the mortality rate fell to 7%. The use of angioplasty increased significantly and surgical intervention rose slightly as the series progressed, and there was a reduction in the incidence of significant bleeding from 15% to 6% (Figure 4.16).

Having achieved satisfactory criteria for selection and a protocol which could be administered with reasonable safety, 52 patients managed by this protocol were followed for a minimum of 4 years[11]. The cause of the occlusion in these patients (Table 4.1) was arterial thrombosis in the majority (64%),

Table 4.1 Causes of occlusion diagnosed by thrombolysis in 52 patients

	%
Arterial thrombosis	64
Embolism	16
Occluded graft	13
Uncertain	7

Table 4.2 Causes of early mortality within 30 days of treatment: 52 patients, seven deaths (14%)

Cause of mortality	Time
1 Peripheral ischaemia	2 d
2 Perforated colonic diverticulum	10 d
3 Bronchopneumonia after amputation	13 d
4 Pulmonary embolism after amputation	3 wk
5 Stroke	3 wk
6 Pneumonia	3 wk
7 Myocardial infarction	4 wk

with both embolism (16%) and graft occlusion (13%) much less common. In a few patients (7%) the cause remained uncertain. After 4 years, 34 patients remained alive, 23 with limb salvage, thrombolysis having been effective initially in 73%. In 6% of these thrombolysis, though effective, produced no clinical benefit. In the majority of survivors, however, the improvement due to thrombolysis was sustained for the 4 years of follow-up. Mortality was 36% in 4 years, nearly half of the deaths occurring within the first 30 days (14%) (Tables 4.2 and 4.3). Amputation was carried out in 12% of patients within 30 days and in 10% during the next 4 years (Table 4.4). Delayed amputation was required for persistent distal occlusions or the progression of distal disease. No death or amputation was caused by the complications of treatment in this series (Table 4.5).

In selected patients the risk of thrombolysis can be reduced to an acceptable level by personal supervision and the use of a strict protocol. It does not work in every case, nor does it always confer clinical benefit when it does work but the low risks of the Guildford protocol make a 'trial of lysis' suitable for many patients with acute ischaemia. In survivors, limb salvage is generally sustained for at least 4 years.

Table 4.3 Causes of later mortality – 30 days – 7 years: 52 patients, 11 deaths (22%)

	Years	Months
1 Pneumonia	0	2
2 Myocardial infarction	1	0
3 Myocardial infarction	1	2
4 Myocardial infarction	2	3
5 Myocardial infarction	2	11
6 Congestive heart failure	3	0
7 Pneumonia	3	6
8 Congestive heart failure	3	10
9 Carcinoma of the colon	4	3
10 Acute renal failure	4	8
11 Multiple strokes	6	10

Total mortality: early and late, 36%.

Table 4.4 Amputation following thrombolysis in 52 patients

Early: up to 30 days   6 (12%)
Late: up to 4 years   5 (10%)

Overall   11 (22%)

Causes of late amputation (30 d to 4 yr)

Progression of distal disease (3)
    0 yr   3 mth
    0 yr   3 mth
    2 yr   8 mth
Embolism from popliteal aneurysm (2)
    0 yr   11 mth
    1 yr   9 mth

Table 4.5 Complications of thrombolysis in 52 patients

MAJOR – 2
1 Neurological defect, CT scan showed intracerebral haemorrhage, full recovery
2 Arterial perforation, vein patch repair

MINOR – 5
1 Allergy (2)
2 Acute confusional state
3 Groin haematoma and abscess
4 Groin haematoma and deep vein thrombosis

COMPLICATIONS OF ANGIOPLASTY AFTER THROMBOLYSIS
1 Vein graft ruptured by attempted angioplasty
2 Atheroma embolized to popliteal artery during angioplasty

Results of other studies

There are now many reports in the literature of thrombolysis in centres where different drugs and techniques of administration have been used successfully. These results have been reviewed in detail by Earnshaw[23]. Of the 1849 patients reported, successful lysis was achieved on average in 62% of patients, with an incidence of minor haemorrhage in about 10%, major haemorrhage in 4% and death associated with the infusion in 3%. The incidence of stroke is very low, although it is the most feared complication, and may be significantly more frequent in regimens employing high-dose techniques of thrombolysis. It may be a particular risk of 'front loading' high-dose techniques but in conventional low-dose regimens it is likely to occur in about 1% of cases.

Long-term results are reported infrequently but other centres using similar regimens have confirmed our experience that, if thrombolysis is associated with limb salvage at 30 days, the patients who survive are unlikely to lose their legs over the next 3 years, although both symptomatic and asymptomatic re-occlusion may occur[57]. Success rates as high as 78% initially and a 2-year cumulative patency rate of 81% after recanalization have been claimed by some[58] and 59% after 5 years by others[59].

Results of thrombolysis in grafts

There is no doubt that thrombolysis can be very effective in the disobliteration of thrombosed vascular grafts, particularly when that thrombosis is recent. Initial success is of the order of 60% but few authors have reported results in the longer term. The available literature suggests that patency has been maintained for at least 1 year in only 30%. It is likely that thrombosis in vein grafts induces permanent intimal damage making re-thrombosis more likely[60]. In synthetic grafts where the re-opened conduit may (at least in theory) be restored to its original state, re-occlusion rates are high[61] and long-term success depends on the correction of the underlying defect causing the thrombosis[62]. Although favourable results have been reported from prophylactic dilatation of strictures and surgical stricturoplasty in stenosed grafts which remain patent, the results of intervention after thrombosis has occurred are much less satisfactory despite successful lysis of thrombus. Graft replacement, or jump grafting in the case of a localized lesion, is to be preferred, particularly if the revision of the original graft would involve the surgical challenge of dissecting and controlling the old anastomosis. It is probably much easier and safer to place a new anastomosis in a virgin field, and whenever possible replacement grafts should be of autogenous vein[63,64].

Conclusion

Thrombolysis is a powerful but potentially dangerous technique which requires careful selection of patients and close adherence to a safe protocol. Each situation poses a different challenge which can only be met by the co-operation of an experienced radiologist and a vascular surgeon, assisted by skilled nurses, radiographers and technicians. There is a significant learning time between being able to use the technique with initial success and being able to select the patient most likely to benefit in the long term and to achieve that result with safety. Every effort should be made to minimize the risk of bleeding and especially stroke. The risk of bleeding is probably an unavoidable consequence of potency. When thrombolysis reveals an underlying arterial defect prompt correction is essential. Thrombolysis has the unique potential to unmask the cause of an acute arterial occlusion and is a valuable addition to the modern integrated management of vascular disease.

References

1. Tillet WS and Garner RL. The fibrinolytic activity of haemolytic streptococci. *J Exp Med* 1933; **58**: 485–502
2. Johnson AJ and McCarty WR. Lysis of artificially induced intravascular clots in man by intravenous infusion of streptokinase. *J Clin Invest* 1959; **38**: 1627–43
3. Chesterman CN, Nash T and Biggs JC. Small vessel thrombosis following vascular injury. Successful treatment with a low-dose intra-arterial infusion of streptokinase. *Br J Surg* 1971; **58**: 582–5
4. Dotter CT, Rosch J, Seaman AJ *et al.* Streptokinase treatment of thromboembolic disease. *Radiology* 1972; **102**: 283–90
5. Dotter CT, Rosch J and Seaman AJ. Selective clot lysis with low dose streptokinase. *Radiology* 1974; **111**: 31–7
6. Gruntzig A and Kumpe DA. Technique of percutaneous transluminal angioplasty with the Gruntzig balloon catheter. *Am J Roentgenol* 1979; **132**: 547–52
7. Katzen BT and van Breda A. Low dose streptokinase in the treatment of arterial occlusions. *Am J Roentgenol* 1981; **136**: 1171–8
8. Hess H, Ingrisch H, Mietaschk A *et al.* Local low-dose thrombolytic therapy of peripheral arterial occlusions. *New Engl J Med* 1982; **307**: 1627–30
9. Walker WJ and Giddings AEB. Low-dose intra-arterial streptokinase: benefit versus risk. *Clin Radiol* 1985; **36**: 345–54
10. Walker WJ and Giddings AEB. A protocol for the safe treatment of acute lower limb ischaemia with intra-arterial streptokinase and surgery. *Br J Surg* 1988; **75**: 1189–92
11. Giddings AEB, Quraishy MS and Walker WJ. Long term results of a single protocol for thrombolysis in acute lower limb ischaemia. *Br J Surg* 1993; **80**: 1262–5
12. Johnson G. Jr. The second generation vascular surgeon. *J Vasc Surg* 1987; **5**: 211–21
13. Mayberry JC, Taylor LM and Porter JM. The epidemiology and natural history of chronic lower-extremity ischemia. In: Wells SA (ed) *Current Problems in Surgery*, XXVIII. Mosby Year Book, London, 1991, pp. 13–28

14. Widmer LK, Biland L and Da Silva A. Risk profile in occlusive peripheral artery disease (OPAD). In: *Proceedings of 13th International Congress of Angiology* (Athens, 9–14 June 1985)
15. Criqui MH, Fronek A, Barrett-Conor E *et al*. The prevalence of peripheral arterial disease in a defined population. *Circulation* 1985; **71**: 510–15
16. Collin J. Avoiding amputation. *Br Med J* 1992; **304**: 856–7
17. Wolfe JHN and Tyrrell MR. Justifying arterial reconstruction to crural vessels – even with a prosthetic graft. *Br J Surg* 1991; **78**: 897–99
18. Anderson JB, Wolinski AP, Wells IP *et al*. The impact of percutaneous transluminal angioplasty on the management of peripheral vascular disease. *Br J Surg* 1986; **73**: 17–19
19. Cheshire NJW, Wolfe JHN, Noone MA *et al*. The economics of femorocrural reconstruction for critical leg ischemia with and without autologous vein. *J Vasc Surg* 1992; **15**: 167–75
20. Kendrick J, Thompson BW, Read RC *et al*. Arterial embolectomy in the leg. Results in a referral hospital. *Am J Surg* 1981; **142**: 739–43
21. Blaisdell FW, Steele M and Allen RE. Management of acute lower extremity arterial ischemia due to embolism and thrombosis. *Surgery* 1978; **84**: 822–34
22. Fogarty TJ, Cranley JJ, Krause RJ *et al*. A method for extraction of arterial emboli and thrombi. *Surg Gynecol Obstet* 1963; **2**: 241–4
23. Earnshaw JJ. Thrombolytic therapy in the management of acute limb ischaemia. *Br J Surg* 1991; **78**: 261–9
24. Abbott WM, Maloney RD, McCabe CC *et al*. Arterial embolism: a 44 year perspective. *Am J Surg* 1982; **143**: 460–4
25. McPhail NV, Fratesi J, Barber GC *et al*. Management of acute thromboembolic limb ischaemia. *Surgery* 1983; **93**: 381–5
26. Jivegard LE, Arfvidsson B, Holm J *et al*. Selective conservative and routine early operative treatment in acute limb ischaemia. *Br J Surg* 1987; **74**: 798–801
27. Berridge DC, Makin GS and Hopkinson BR. Local low dose intra-arterial thrombolytic therapy: the risk of stroke or major haemorrhage. *Br J Surg* 1989; **76**: 1230–3
28. Mann RD. Unlicensed medicines and the use of drugs in unlicensed indications. In: Goldberg A, Dodds-Smith I (ed) *Pharmaceutical Medicine and the Law*. Royal College of Physicians, London, 1991; pp. 103–10
29. O'Brien TS, Thomas H, Crow A *et al*. Calf vessel preservation in peripheral vascular disease – angiography versus pulse generated run-off. *Eur J Vasc Surg* 1993; **7**: 177–9
30. Bird D, Giddings AEB and Jones SM. Non-clostridial gas gangrene in the diabetic lower limb. *Diabetologia* 1977; **13**: 373–6
31. Joint Working Party of the Royal College of Radiologists and the The Royal College of Anaesthetists. *Sedation and Anaesthesia in Radiology*. London, 1992
32. Bell WR and Meek AG. Guidelines for the use of thrombolytic agents. *New Engl J Med* 1979; **301**: 1266–70
33. ISIS-2 (Second International Study of Infarct Survival) Collaborative Group. Randomised trial of intravenous streptokinase, oral aspirin, both, or neither among 17 187 cases of suspected acute myocardial infarction. *Lancet* 1988; **ii**: 349–60
34. McGarth KG and Patterson R. Anaphylactic reactivity to streptokinase. *JAMA* 1984; **252**: 1314–7
35. Coon WW and Willis PW 3rd. Haemorrhagic complications of anticoagulant treatment. *Arch Int Med* 1974; **133**: 386–92
36. Buckenham TM, George CD, Chester JF *et al*. Accelerated thrombolysis using pulsed intra-thrombus recombinant human tissue type plasminogen activator (rt-PA). *Eur J Vasc Surg* 1992; **6**: 237–40
37. Beard JD, Nyamekye I, Earnshaw JJ *et al*. Intraoperative streptokinase: a useful adjunct to balloon-catheter embolectomy. *Br J Surg* 1993; **80**: 21–4
38. Harris PL. Vein graft surveillance – all part of the service. *Br J Surg* 1992; **79**: 97–8
39. Franks PJ, Sian M, Kenchington GF *et al*. Aspirin usage and its influence on femoropopliteal vein graft patency. *Eur J Vasc Surg* 1992; **6**: 185–8
40. Browse DJ, Torrie EPH and Galland RB. Low-dose intra-arterial thrombolysis in the treatment of occluded vascular grafts. *Br J Surg* 1992; **79**: 86–8

41. Dawson I, van Bockel JH, Brand R *et al.* Popliteal artery aneurysms. Long-term follow-up of aneurysmal disease and results of surgical treatment. *J Vasc Surg* 1991; **13**: 398–407
42. Downing R, Grimley RP, Ashton F *et al.* Problems in diagnosis of popliteal aneurysms. *J Roy Soc Med* 1985; **78**: 440–4
43. Lancashire MJR, Torrie EPH and Galland RB. Popliteal aneurysms identified by intra-arterial streptokinase: a changing pattern of presentation. *Br J Surg* 1990; **77**: 1388–90
44. Quraishy MS and Giddings AEB. Treatment of asymptomatic popliteal aneurysm: protection at a price. *Br J Surg* 1992; **79**: 731–2
45. Shortell CK, DeWeese JA, Ouriel K *et al.* Popliteal artery aneurysms: a 25-year surgical experience. *J Vasc Surg* 1991; **14**: 771–9
46. Sciolaro C, Hunter GC, McIntyre KE *et al.* Thrombectomy and isolated limb perfusion with urokinase in the treatment of phlegmasia cerulea dolens. *Cardiovasc Surg* 1993; **1**: 56–60
47. Royston D. High-dose aprotinin therapy: a review of the first five years' experience. *J Cardiothor Vasc Anesth* 1992; **6**: 76–100
48. Abu-Yousef MM, Wiese JA and Shamma AR. The 'to-and-fro' sign: duplex Doppler evidence of femoral artery pseudoaneurysm. *Am J Roentgenol* 1988; **150**: 632–4
49. Kram HB, Schwartz C and Veith FJ. Open techniques for removal of intraarterial sheath after urokinase infusion in patients undergoing heparinization. *J Vasc Surg* 1992; **16**: 937–8
50. Kresowik TF, Khoury MD, Miller BV *et al.* A prospective study of the incidence and natural history of femoral vascular complications after percutaneous transluminal coronary angioplasty. *J. Vasc Surg* 1991; **13**: 328–36
51. Feld R, Patton GM, Carabasi RA *et al.* Treatment of iatrogenic femoral artery injuries with ultrasound-guided compression. *J Vasc Surg* 1992; **16**: 832–40
52. Wilkins DC, Bliss BP and Wells IP. Conservative management of asymptomatic popliteal aneurysm. *Br J Surg* 1992; **79**: 710
53. Galland RB, Earnshaw JJ, Baird RN *et al.* Acute limb deterioration during intra-arterial thrombolysis. *Br J Surg.* 1993; **80**: 1118–20
54. Berridge DC, Gregson RHS, Makin GS *et al.* Tissue plasminogen activator in peripheral arterial thrombolysis. *Br J Surg* 1990; **77**: 179–82
55. Schulman S, Lockner D, Grandqvist S *et al.* A comparative randomized trial of low-dose versus high-dose streptokinase in deep vein thrombosis of the thigh. *Thromb Haemost* 1984; **51**: 261–5
56. Sarin S, Shami SK, Cheatle TR *et al.* When do vascular surgeons prescribe antiplatelet therapy? Current attitudes. *Eur J Vasc Surg* 1993; **7**: 6–13
57. Lonsdale RJ, Whitaker SC, Berridge DC *et al.* Peripheral arterial thrombolysis: intermediate term results. *Br J Surg* 1993; **80**: 592–5
58. Lammer J, Pilger E, Neumayer K *et al.* Intraarterial fibrinolysis: long-term results. *Radiology* 1986; **161**: 159–63
59. Hess H. Mietaschk A and Bruckl R. Peripheral arterial occlusions: a 6-year experience with local low-dose thrombolytic therapy. *Radiology* 1987; **163**: 753–8
60. Belkin M, Donaldson MC, Whittemore AD *et al.* Observations on the use of thrombolytic agents for thrombotic occlusion of infrainguinal vein grafts. *J Vasc Surg* 1990; **11**: 289–96
61. Guest P and Buckenham T. Thrombolysis of the occluded prosthetic graft with tissue-type plasminogen activator – technique, results and problems in 23 patients. *Clin Radiol* 1992; **46**: 381–6
62. Gardiner GA, Harrington DP, Koltun W *et al.* Salvage of occluded arterial bypass grafts by means of thrombolysis. *J Vasc Surg* 1989; **9**: 426–31
63. Sullivan KL, Gardiner GA, Kandarpa K *et al.* Efficacy of thrombolysis in infrainguinal bypass grafts. *Circulation* 1991; **83**: 199–205
64. Edwards JE, Taylor LM and Porter JM. Treatment of failed lower extremity bypass grafts with new autogenous vein bypass grafting. *J Vasc Surg* 1990; **11**: 136–45

Chapter 5

Radiological techniques in thrombolysis

R. H. S. Gregson

The basic technique

Diagnostic arteriography

Urgent or emergency arteriography is necessary in most patients presenting with acute critical lower limb arterial ischaemia. It is difficult to distinguish clinically between an arterial thrombosis and an arterial embolus in a patient who is likely to have underlying atherosclerosis in their lower limb vessels (Figure 5.1).

It is best to perform the diagnostic arteriography by catheterizing the contralateral femoral artery in the normal leg with a 4 or 5F pigtail catheter (Table 5.1). The arteriography helps to decide the management of the patient by outlining the site and length of the occlusion, the patency of the distal vessels and the state of the lower limb arteries.

With both the clinical and the radiological information, a joint decision between the vascular surgeon and radiologist can then be made as to whether intra-arterial thrombolysis is appropriate for the treatment of this acute arterial occlusion. If it is, then a catheter needs to be positioned immediately for the delivery of the thrombolytic infusion.

Catheter position for short arterial occlusions

For short arterial occlusions (less than 10–15 cm in length) in the common or external iliac artery, the common femoral artery or the proximal superficial femoral artery, the pigtail catheter is exchanged for a 4 or 5F gauge side-winder or cobra catheter with an end hole and two side holes, as access to the vascular system is already available following the diagnostic arteriography via the contra-lateral femoral artery (Table 5.2). The side-winder or cobra catheter is positioned across the aortic bifurcation with its tip 2–3 cm into the occlusion, secured to the skin by a clear plastic adhesive dressing and flushed with 5000 units of heparin. The thrombolytic drug infusion regimen using either streptokinase, urokinase or tissue plasminogen activator can then be started (Figure 5.2).

For short arterial occlusions in the distal superficial femoral or popliteal arteries the tip of a 4 or 5F gauge straight catheter with an end hole and several side holes can be positioned within the thrombus using a similar

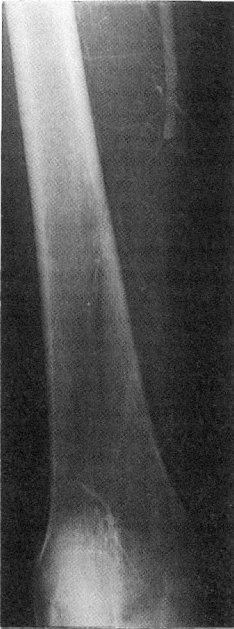

Figure 5.1 Superficial femoral artery occlusion: but is it embolus or thrombus?

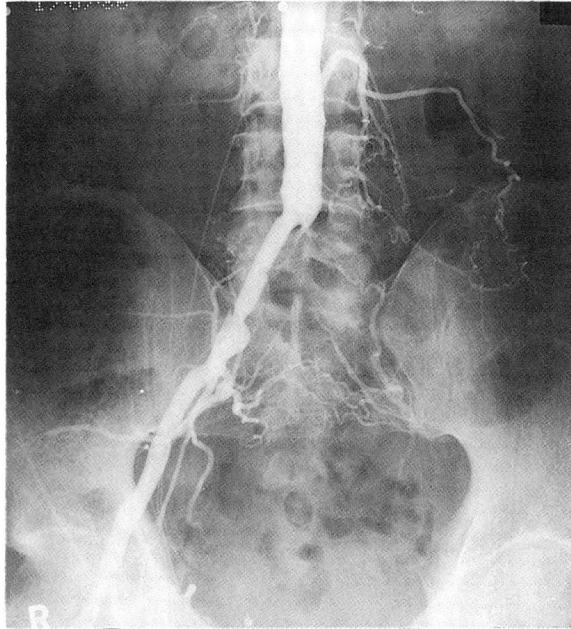

(a)

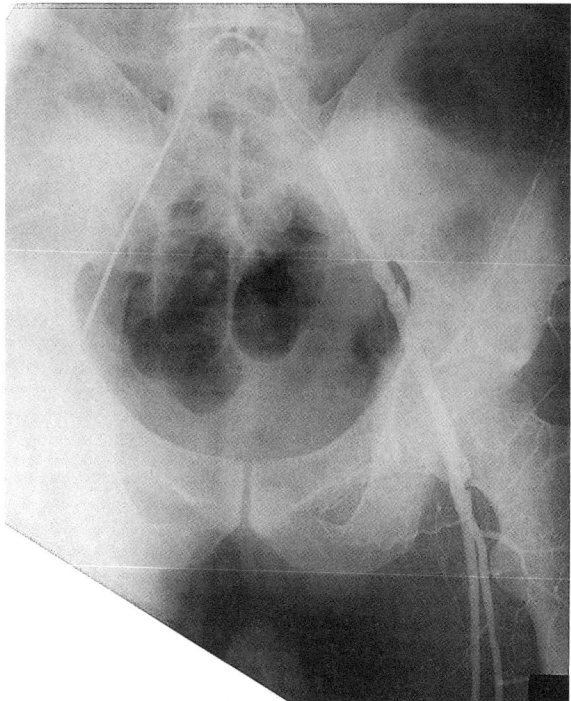

Figure 5.2 Retrograde technique. (a) Left common iliac artery thrombosis extending into common femoral artery. (b) Successful lysis using 7F side-winder catheter across aortic bifurcation

(b)

Table 5.1 Equipment required for diagnostic arteriography

1. Thin-walled 19 gauge one-part needle or 18 gauge two-part needle
2. 0.89 mm (0.035 in) Teflon-coated 150 cm guidewire with a 3 mm J-shaped tip
3. 4 or 5F gauge 100 cm pigtail catheter with an end hole and multiple side holes near the tip
4. Low osmolar non-ionic contrast medium containing 300–370 mg I/ml for conventional angiography or 150–200 mg I/ml for digital subtraction angiography

Table 5.2 Equipment required for thrombolysis (cross-over technique using retrograde catheterization of femoral artery following diagnostic arteriography via initial arterial puncture)

1. 0.89 mm (0.035 in) Teflon-coated 150 cm guidewire with a 3 mm J-shaped tip
2. 5 or 6F gauge sheath with a haemostatic valve and side port for flushing
3. 5F gauge 100 cm side-winder or 50 cm cobra catheter with an end hole and two side holes near the tip
4. 0.89 mm (0.035 in) hydrophilic-coated 150 cm guidewire with a straight or angled tip
5. 0.89 mm (0.035 in) Teflon-coated heavy duty 150 cm guidewire with a straight or 1.5 mm J-shaped tip
6. 5F gauge 100 cm straight catheter with an end hole and several side holes near the tip

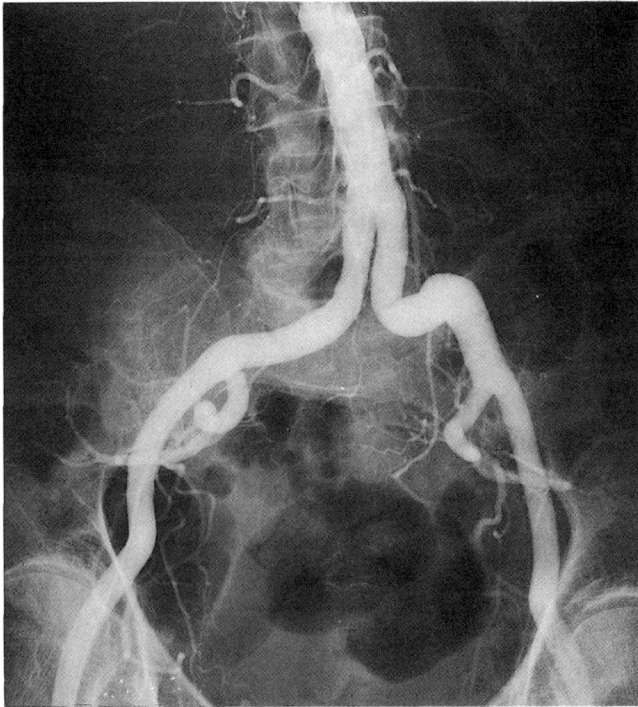

Figure 5.3 Aortic bifurcation with acute angle and tortuous iliac arteries. Cross-over technique may be difficult

Table 5.3 Equipment required for thrombolysis (direct technique using antegrade catheterization of femoral artery following diagnostic arteriography via another arterial puncture)

1. Thin-walled 19 gauge one-part needle or 18 gauge two-part needle
2. 0.89 mm (0.035 in) Teflon-coated 150 cm guidewire with a straight tip
3. 5 or 6F gauge sheath with a haemostatic valve and side port for flushing
4. 0.89 mm (0.035 in) hydrophilic-coated 150 cm guidewire with a straight or angled tip
5. 4 or 5F gauge 100 cm straight catheter with an end hole and several side holes near the tip

Table 5.4 Equipment required for angioplasty (following thrombolysis via the sheath)

1. 0.89 mm (0.035 in) Teflon-coated 150 cm guidewire with a straight or 3 mm J-shaped tip
2. 0.89 mm (0.035 in) Teflon-coated exchange 250 cm guidewire with a straight tip
3. 5 or 6F gauge 100 cm angioplasty catheter with a high pressure balloon 4–10 mm in diameter
4. 0.45 mm (0.018 in) safety 150 cm guidewire with a straight tip

technique for crossing the aortic bifurcation (Table 5.2). The advantage of this aortic bifurcation cross-over technique is that it only produces one arterial puncture site. However, it is not always easy to do, particularly if the iliac arteries are either tortuous or markedly atheromatous and if the aortic bifurcation has a narrow, acute angle (Figure 5.3). Therefore for short occlusions in the distal superficial femoral, popliteal or tibial arteries the tip of a 4 or 5F gauge straight catheter should be positioned 2–3 cm into the occlusion following antegrade catheterization of the ipsi-lateral femoral artery in the ischaemic leg (Figure 5.4 and Table 5.3). The advantage of this direct antegrade technique is that it makes a subsequent angioplasty very much easier to perform. However, it produces a second arterial puncture site which increases the risk of groin haematoma.

Angioplasty

When complete lysis of thrombus has been achieved the patient returns to the X-ray suite for further arteriography, which helps to decide on further management by revealing any underlying residual arterial stenosis, the presence of peri-catheter thrombus or distal embolic thrombus and the state of the lower limb arteries.

If arteriography shows that the arteries are now patent, the infusion catheter is removed and haemostasis in the groin achieved by direct pressure at the puncture site. If there is a significant residual arterial stenosis, percutaneous transluminal angioplasty using a 5F gauge catheter with a high pressure balloon should be performed at the time, after 2000–5000 units heparin. Check angiography is performed to ensure adequate angioplasty and then the balloon catheter is removed as above (Figure 5.5 and Table 5.4).

The desired result from thrombolysis of a critically ischaemic leg is limb salvage without any complications, but the ideal result is a useful leg with no persisting ischaemia clinically and patent vessels radiologically. Thrombolysis is not always successful and if no lysis of the thrombus has occurred within 12–24 hours the infusion catheter should be removed. As long as there

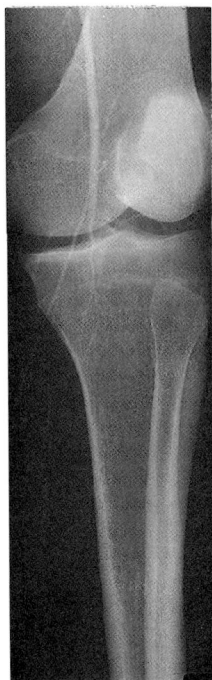

(a)

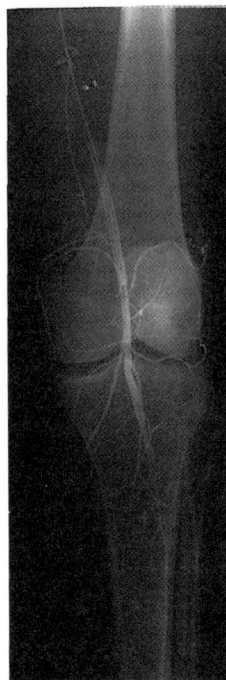

(b)

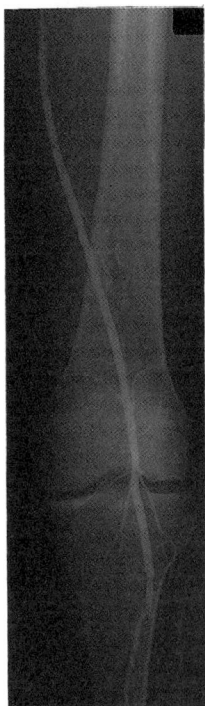

(c)

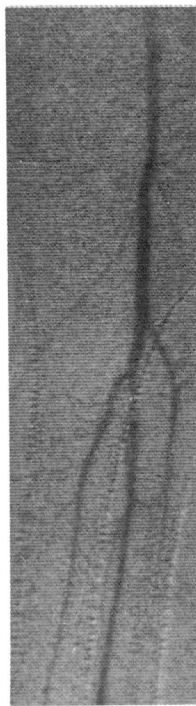

(d)

Figure 5.4 Antegrade thrombolysis.
(a) Popliteal artery embolus.
(b) Antegrade lysis with 4F catheter
inserted into thrombus. (Note
pericatheter thrombosis.) (c) After
successful thrombolysis. (d) Result
1 month later

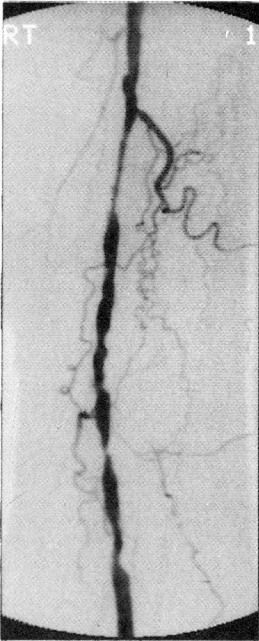

(a)

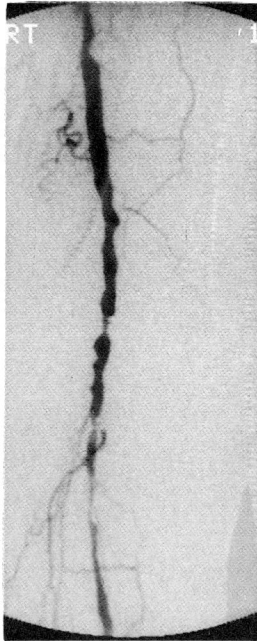

(b)

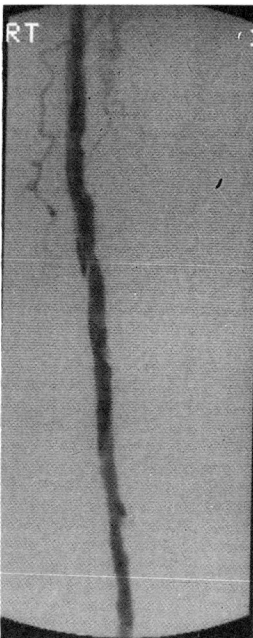

(c)

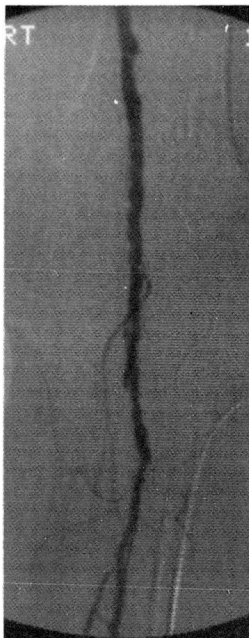

(d)

Figure 5.5 Angioplasty.
(a), (b) After successful lysis of the
superficial femoral artery occlusion,
multiple residual stenoses are
revealed. (c), (d). After successful
angioplasties

is continuing arteriographic evidence of lysis of the thrombus, without any clinical deterioration of the limb or any haemorrhagic complications, thrombolysis can be successfully continued for up to 80–100 hours!

Modifications for short occlusions

There are several simple modifications to this basic radiological technique, which may also be helpful in thrombolytic therapy.

Fragmentation of the thrombus

This can be produced by advancing a guidewire beyond the tip of the catheter into the occlusion. Gentle manipulation of the guidewire fragments the thrombus and this increases the surface area for the thrombolytic drug to act upon[1]. The guidewire sometimes passes completely through the occlusion into a patent distal vessel during the manipulation.

Use of a vascular sheath

This produces less discomfort for the patient during catheter manipulation, makes the completion angioplasty easier for the radiologist to perform and allows further vascular access if the catheter is damaged or removed by the patient. Heparin or thrombolytic solution can also be infused through the sheath in order to prevent peri-catheter thrombosis. However, the use of a sheath within a narrow artery predisposes to peri-sheath thrombosis!

Catheter tip position above the occlusion

This is not an effective position for the catheter during thrombolysis, but may lead to softening of the proximal end of the occlusion and allow subsequent positioning of the tip of the catheter within the thrombus, if this had not been possible initially (Figure 5.6).[2]

Modifications for long occlusions

There are two modifications to the basic radiological technique for short arterial occlusions, which are required in the treatment of long arterial occlusions (more than 20–30 cm in length) by thrombolytic therapy.

Advancing the catheter

With the tip of the infusion catheter positioned 2–3 cm into a long 20–30 cm occlusion, the thrombolytic drug will only produce lysis of the proximal 10 cm of thrombus. Therefore in order to lyse the distal 20 cm of thrombus, the catheter needs to be advanced so that its tip is once again positioned within the residual thrombus[3]. This will need to be done once more in order

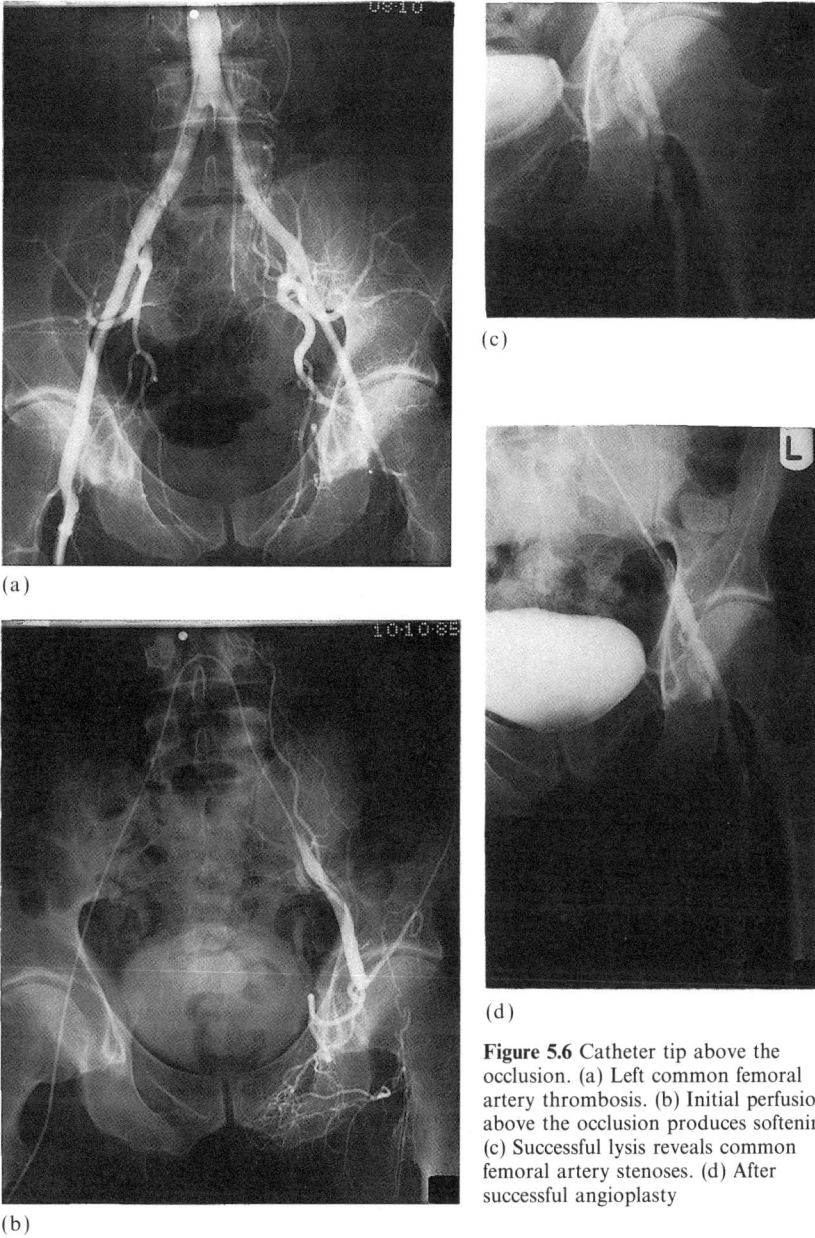

(a)

(b)

(c)

(d)

Figure 5.6 Catheter tip above the occlusion. (a) Left common femoral artery thrombosis. (b) Initial perfusion above the occlusion produces softening. (c) Successful lysis reveals common femoral artery stenoses. (d) After successful angioplasty

to lyse the final 10 cm of thrombus and obviously several times for occlusions up to 50–60 cm in length.

The disadvantages of this modification are that the re-positioning has to be done in the angiography room and that a new sterile catheter has to be used, as a 10 cm length of the unsterile infusion catheter cannot be advanced over a guidewire and into the artery.

(a)

(b)

(c)

(d)

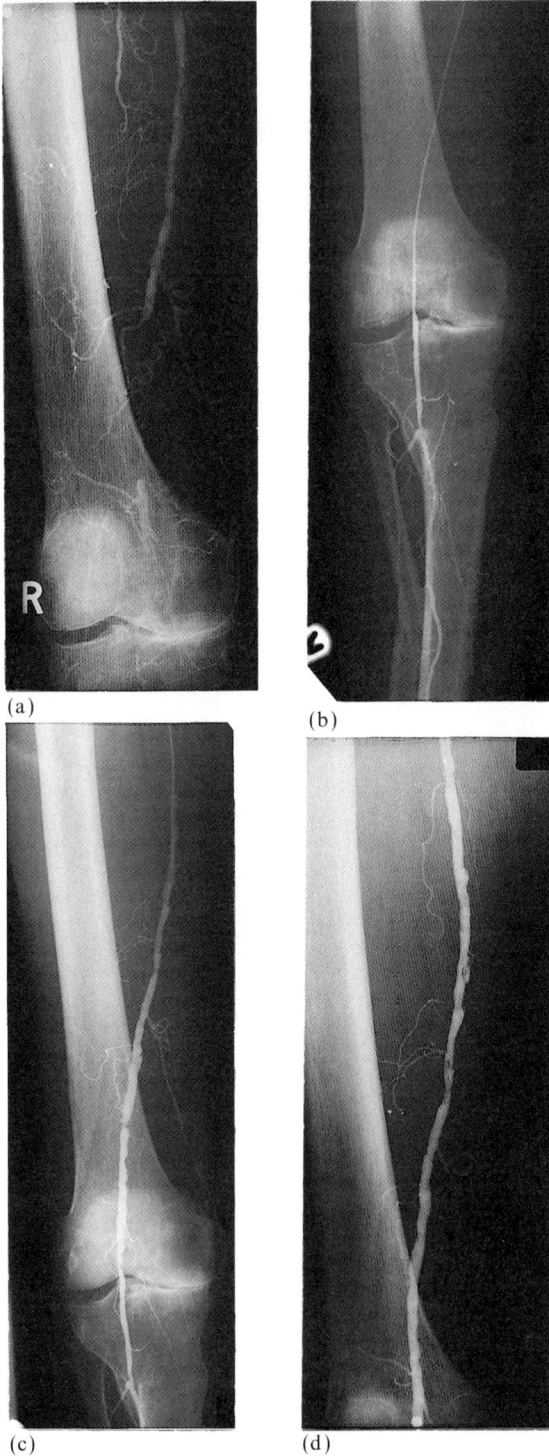

Figure 5.7 Catheter withdrawal technique. (a) A long occlusion from distal superficial femoral artery extending into tibial vessels. (b) Antegrade approach, catheter tip positioned at distal end of occlusion and withdrawn as distal vessels lysed. (c) Successful recanalization of superficial femoral artery reveals underlying stenosis. (d) After successful angioplasty

Withdrawing the catheter

With the tip of the infusion catheter positioned 18–20 cm into a long 30 cm occlusion, the thrombolytic drug will only produce lysis of the distal 10 cm of thrombus. Therefore in order to lyse the proximal 20 cm of thrombus, the catheter needs to be withdrawn so that its tip is once again positioned within the remaining thrombus. This will also need to be done once more in order to lyse the final 10 cm of thrombus (Figure 5.7). The disadvantage of this modification is that it can be difficult to position the infusion catheter near the distal end of occlusions up to 50–60 cm in length. However, the advantages of this modification, which was described by Earnshaw *et al.*[4], are that the re-positioning can be done on the ward and that once the distal vessels are patent, perfusion of the ischaemic leg is improved due to blood flow from collateral vessels. A surgical by-pass graft also becomes a treatment option once the distal vessels are patent.

Bedside assessment of distal patency is possible without recourse to angiography. Easy aspiration of bright red arterial blood up the infusion catheter implies distal vessel patency so the catheter can be withdrawn a few centimetres at more frequent intervals and lysis speeded up.

Developments in radiological technique

During the 1980s there have been a large number of series published on the treatment of acute lower limb arterial ischaemia by low-dose intra-arterial thrombolytic therapy, using streptokinase at a dose of 5000–10 000 units/h[5–10]. Increasing use of both urokinase, at a dose of 20 000–50 000 units/h[1,11,12], and t-PA, at a dose of 0.5–2 mg/h[13–15], has been apparent over the last 5 years.

Successful lysis of the thrombus occurs in over 60% of patients (but ranges from 40% to 80% in different series) using low-dose streptokinase and this results in limb salvage in 50–70% of patients. A similar range for successful lysis can be achieved by using low-dose urokinase, but low-dose t-PA reportedly produces a higher successful lysis rate of 80–100%[16]. Low-dose t-PA (0.5 mg/h) with a lysis rate of 100% and a limb salvage rate of 80% has been shown to be superior to low-dose streptokinase (5000 units/h) with a lysis rate of 80% and a limb salvage rate of 60% in a small randomized trial of 40 patients, published by Berridge *et al.*[17].

The duration of the infusion or the time to lysis of the thrombus is dependent upon the length of the arterial occlusion and the dose of the fibrinolytic drug used in the infusion. The mean infusion times for low-dose streptokinase, urokinase and t-PA are between 20 and 30 hours in most series, but range from 15 to 40 hours[16].

Improvements in the thrombolytic treatment of acute arterial ischaemia of the lower limb could in theory be made by:

1. Decreasing the time to lysis of the thrombus.
2. Increasing the rate of successful lysis of the thrombus.
3. Reducing the incidence of haemorrhagic complications.

The result of these improvements should be a higher rate of limb salvage, but how can this be achieved in practice? Developments in radiological

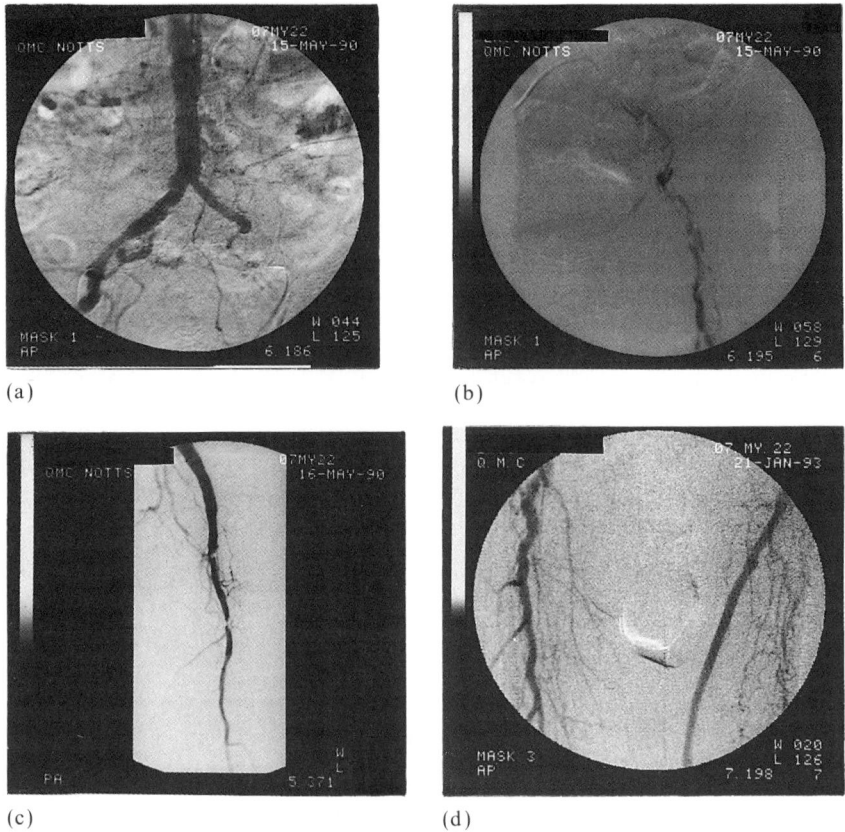

(a)

(b)

(c)

(d)

Figure 5.8 Combination of lysis and surgery. (a)Left common iliac artery occlusion.
(b) Thrombolysis using contra-lateral technique and 5F side-winder catheter. (c) Successful
thrombolysis restores femoral pulse. The residual stenoses are shown. (d) Left
femoro-popliteal graft later required to revascularize the ischaemic foot

techniques such as high-dose infusion regimens and new infusion catheters
certainly provide part of the answer.

Improved patient selection, advances in the concept of combined surgical
and thrombolytic treatment (Figure 5.8) and new, more effective fibrinolytic
drugs also provide part of the answer.

High-dose infusion and bolus regimens (accelerated thrombolysis)

Accelerating thrombolysis offers the advantage of reducing the duration of
limb ischaemia and tissue damage. This may increase the indications of
thrombolysis to include patients with more severe acute leg ischaemia. Most
accelerated techniques, however, require larger doses of thrombolytic drugs
which potentially increases the risk of side-effects such as haemorrhage or
distal embolization.

Over the last 10 years there have also been a small number of series published advocating the treatment of acute arterial ischaemia of the lower limb by high-dose intra-arterial thrombolytic therapy using streptokinase, urokinase and t-PA.

High-dose streptokinase

The first report of high-dose streptokinase with a catheter advancement technique was produced by Hess *et al* in 1982 in 136 patients[3]. They described how the tip of a catheter was placed about 1 cm into the occlusion. 1000–3000 units of streptokinase in 1–3 ml of normal saline was then injected into the thrombus. After 5–15 minutes the catheter was advanced a little, if there was some lysis of thrombus, and a further bolus of streptokinase injected. This process was repeated until the tip of the catheter reached the patent lumen of the artery distally. Residual stenotic lesions were then treated by angioplasty. Heparin was not given during the procedure. Lysis of the thrombus was achieved in 69% of patients with a lysis time of only 1–5 hours! However, there was an early re-occlusion rate of 18% with only 51% of patients having a patent arterial segment at 15 days. There were no major haemorrhagic complications recorded, but groin haematoma occurred in 2% of patients. This technique has subsequently been modified by the group so that the tip of the catheter is initially placed above the occlusion, because sub-intimal dissection of the catheter at the origin of the occlusion or failure to enter the occlusion occurred in 28% of patients in their first series. They now inject 1000 units of streptokinase in 2 ml of normal saline (or 3000 units of urokinase) on three occasions at intervals of 3 minutes to soften the thrombus initially. The catheter is then advanced into the occlusion and 1000 units of streptokinase in 2 ml of normal saline is injected every 3 minutes (or at 2-minute intervals for long occlusions). The catheter is advanced as lysis of the thrombus occurs, as before. The dose of streptokinase being used therefore is 20 000–30 000 units/h. The hospital mortality rate of 1.6% with an amputation rate of 2% in this series totalling 564 patients[2], are both very impressive, although the overall lysis rate remains 51%.

High-dose urokinase

McNamara and Fischer used a high dose of urokinase with a catheter advancement technique in 93 patients[18]. They initially advanced a guidewire through the thrombus to see whether it was soft or well organized. The tip of a catheter was then advanced 2 cm into the occlusion and urokinase infused at a dose of 4000 units/min (i.e. 240 000 units/h in 96 ml of fluid). After 2 hours the catheter was advanced distally if there had been some lysis of thrombus and urokinase was infused again at a dose of 4000 units/min for a further 2 hours. When there was a patent channel through the lysing thrombus the catheter was withdrawn proximally and urokinase infused again but at a reduced dose of 1000 units/min for 4–8 hours. Angioplasty was then performed if necessary. Heparin at a dose of 1000 units/h was given intravenously during the procedure. Lysis of the thrombus was achieved in 75% of patients with an average duration of 18 hours. Major haemorrhage requiring transfusion occurred in 4% of patients and groin haematoma in

3%. The hospital mortality rate and amputation rate have not been recorded in this series totalling 150 patients[19], but the results are similar and suggest that there is no difference between the use of low- and high-dose urokinase infusion regimens[20], which is surprising as both high-dose streptokinase and t-PA do produce a significant reduction in the lysis time.

Cragg et al[21] confirmed this finding in a randomized trial of 63 patients with both native arterial and graft occlusions, treated with low-dose urokinase (50 000 units/h) or high-dose urokinase (250 000 units/h for 4 hours and then 125 000 units/h). They showed that there was no significant difference between the groups in terms of clinically successful lysis, which ranged from 65% to 85%, and duration of the infusion, which ranged from 22 to 35 hours.

High-dose t-PA

Verstraete et al. used a high dose of t-PA with a catheter advancement technique in 66 patients[22]. They also described how the tip of a catheter was advanced into the proximal part of the occlusion and t-PA infused at a dose of 10 mg/h in 20 ml of normal saline. The catheter was advanced at hourly intervals as the thrombus lysed and angioplasty was performed as residual arterial stenoses were revealed. Heparinization during the procedure was produced by an intra-arterial bolus of 2500–5000 units, an intra-arterial infusion of 400 units/h or an intravenous infusion of 1000 units/h. t-PA was also infused more slowly in some patients in this pilot study at doses of 3 and 5 mg/h. Lysis of the thrombus was achieved in 86% of patients receiving 10 mg/h, but the re-thrombosis rate of 10% reduced this to 76% at 7 days. Major haemorrhage requiring transfusion occurred in 4% of patients, but groin haematoma occurred in 16%. Lysis of the thrombus was also achieved in 94% of patients receiving doses of 3 and 5 mg/h but was reduced by re-thrombosis to 81% at 7 days. There were no major haemorrhagic complications recorded, but groin haematoma occurred in 37% of these patients.

Graor et al[23] treated 33 patients with t-PA using doses of 0.05 and 0.1 mg/kg/h (i.e. about 3–10 mg/h) and produced lysis of thrombus in 97% of patients with a mean lysis time of less than 4 hours. Major haemorrhage requiring transfusion occurred in 3% of patients and groin haematoma in 12%. This group publish consistently impressive results with t-PA[24].

Meyerovitz et al.[25] performed a small randomized trial of 32 patients with both native arterial and graft occlusions, treated with high-dose t-PA (an initial 10 mg bolus followed by an infusion of 5 mg/h up to 24 hours) or high-dose urokinase (an initial 60 000 units bolus followed by an infusion of 240 000 units/h for 2 hours, 120 000 units/h for 2 hours and then 60 000 units/h up to 20 hours). Accelerated lysis with t-PA was superior to urokinase in terms of the duration of lysis, although the rate of haemorrhagic complications was higher with t-PA, but this was not statistically significant.

In the method used by Meyerovitz, the initial bolus of the thrombolytic drug (10 mg t-PA or 60 000 units urokinase) was delivered throughout the thrombus by a continuous injection as the tip of the infusion catheter was gradually withdrawn from the distal end of the occlusion to the proximal end over several seconds. The infusion of the thrombolytic drug was then started from the proximal end of the occlusion. This technique is called lacing the thrombus and increases the surface area for the thrombolytic drug's action. It depends upon being able to position the tip of the catheter at the distal end of the occlusion initially. Lacing is a simple method of accelerating thrombolysis and deserves more widespread use.

Recently Buckenham et al.[26] have also used high-dose t-PA in a bolus and infusion technique in 20 patients with both graft and native arterial occlusions. They used three 5 mg boluses injected at 10-minute intervals into the thrombus, followed by an infusion of 0.05 mg/kg/h if necessary with continued advancement of the catheter. This produced lysis of thrombus in 100% of patients with a mean lysis time of 109 minutes. Haemorrhagic complications occurred in 15% of patients. Braithwaite et al.[27] only produced lysis of thrombus in 74% of patients with a mean lysis time of 7 hours in 33 patients with native arterial occlusions using a similar technique.

New infusion catheters

The catheters used to deliver the infusion of the thrombolytic drug are normally 4 or 5F gauge catheters with either an end hole alone or an end hole with several side holes near the tip. 6 or 7F gauge catheters are also occasionally used.

For occlusions in small narrow arteries such as the anterior and posterior tibial arteries or the common peroneal artery it is best to use either a 2F gauge catheter or a guidewire with an injection lumen in a co-axial system through a 5F gauge catheter and a vascular sheath (Figure 5.9). A 2 or 3F gauge catheter in a co-axial system with a 5 or 6F gauge catheter can also be used to lace thrombus with a thrombolytic drug prior to starting the main infusion.

A co-axial system incorporating a vascular sheath can also be used to deliver a thrombolytic drug infusion at three different levels:

1. From the tip of the 2F gauge catheter or guidewire with an injection lumen into distal thrombus.
2. From the tip of the 5F gauge catheter into proximal thrombus.
3. From the tip of the vascular sheath into the patent arterial lumen to prevent peri-catheter thrombosis.

Multi-level infusions are suitable for patients with either a single long occlusion or two short occlusions in the same leg, because they increase the surface area for the thrombolytic drug's action.

Occlusions of up to 20 cm in length can also be treated by a multi-level infusion from a single 5F catheter with four side holes from four independent infusion channels within the catheter. Multiple side hole catheters can be tailored to the length of the occlusion with the four holes close together for a catheter with an infusion length of 4 cm and far apart for a catheter with an infusion length of 18 cm. The catheter is positioned with the side holes at the centre of an occlusion.

The use of a 7F catheter with two side holes between an angioplasty balloon at the tip of the catheter and another more proximal angioplasty balloon allows thrombolysis to be performed in an enclosed segment of the

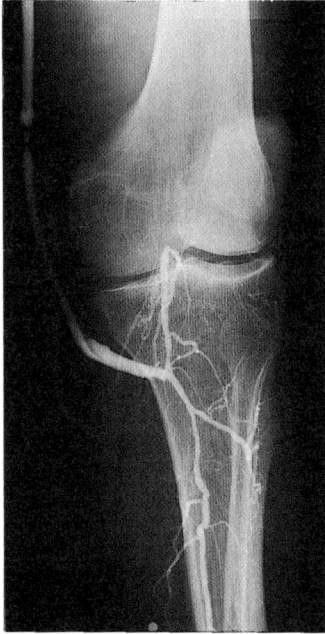

(a)

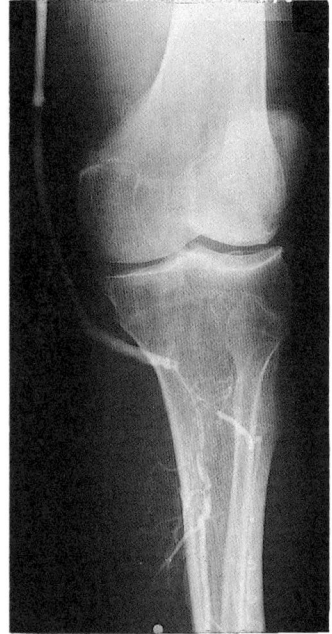

(b)

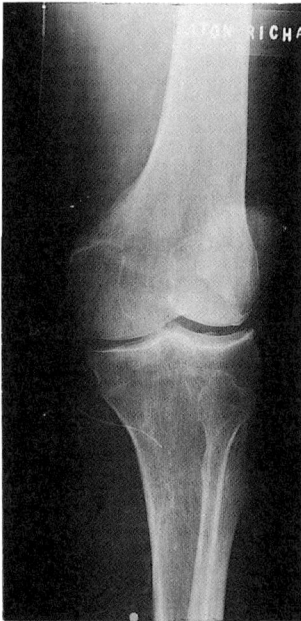

(c)

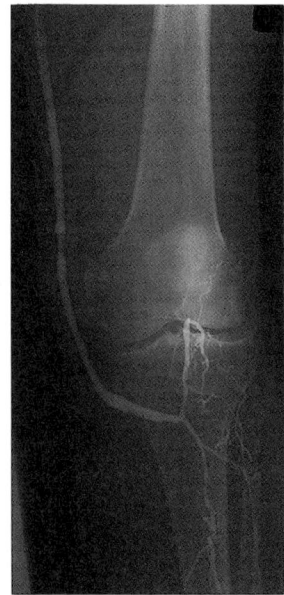

(d)

Figure 5.9 (a) Femoro-popliteal vein graft stenosis (same patient as in Figure 5.8 but 3 years later). (b) Embolic occlusion in popliteal and tibial arteries following angioplasty.
(c) Co-axial technique. Distal thrombolysis using infusion guidewire. (d) After successful clearance of run-off vessels

femoro-popliteal artery, following recanalization angioplasty of chronic occlusions from 1 to 15 cm in length in order to prevent early re-thrombosis. This technique could easily be adapted for acute occlusions as well[28].

Pulsed spray thrombolysis

Undoubtedly the most exciting recent development in thrombolysis is the technique of pulsed spray pharmaco-mechanical thrombolysis. This technique was described by Bookstein *et al.*[29] in 41 patients. It involves small pulses of a high dose of urokinase being injected as a spray throughout the thrombus via the 5F infusion catheter, which has multiple side holes. The end hole of the catheter must be occluded by a special tip occluding guidewire during the lysis treatment in order to produce the spray effect (Figure 5.10). The number of side holes or slits ranges from 10 to 150 and these are equally spaced over a length of catheter which varies from 4 to 30 cm. As above, the catheter is tailored to the length of the occlusion, so that the side holes or slits are within the thrombus (Figure 5.11).

Each pulse consists of 5000 units of urokinase in 0.2 ml of sterile water, which is injected forcefully by a 1 ml syringe from a solution containing 25 000 units/ml every 15–30 seconds. About 150 000 units of urokinase are initially delivered in 10–20 minutes. The concentration of the solution of urokinase is then diluted to 5000–10 000 units/ml and an additional 50 000 units of urokinase are injected either as pulses or a continuous infusion over the next 1–2 hours, until lysis is complete.

A bolus of 3000–5000 units of heparin is given at the start of the thrombolysis and a further 3000–5000 units of heparin are given before angioplasty with an additional 1000–2000 units/h for procedures lasting more than 1 hour.

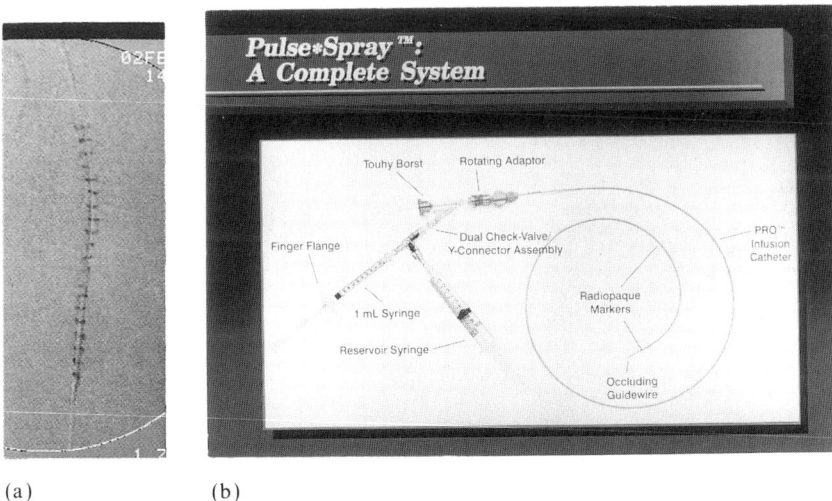

(a)   (b)

Figure 5.10 (a) Angiogram showing pulsed spray effect of contrast medium injected through a 5F catheter with a tip occluding guidewire in position. (b) Pulse spray thrombolytic system (E-Z-EM Ltd)

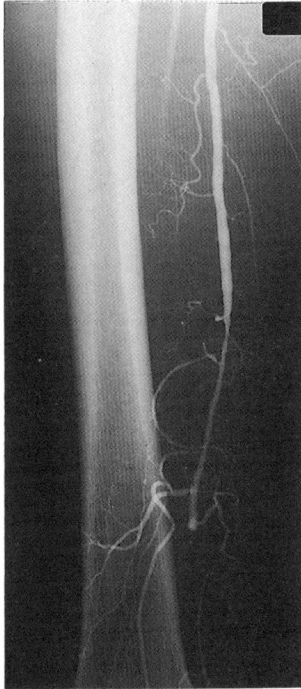

(a)

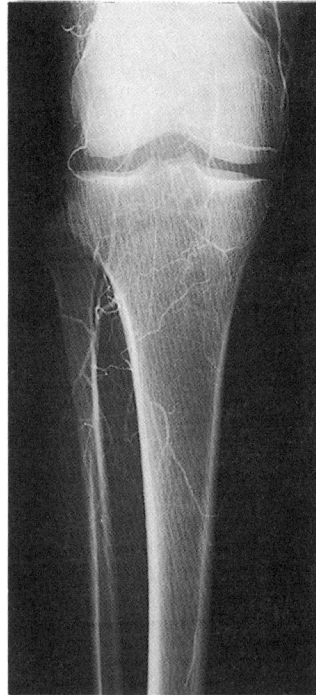

(b)

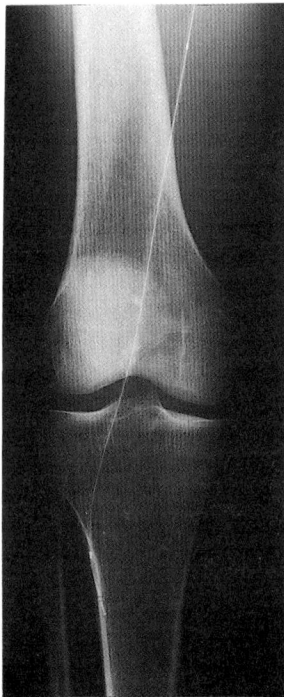

(c)

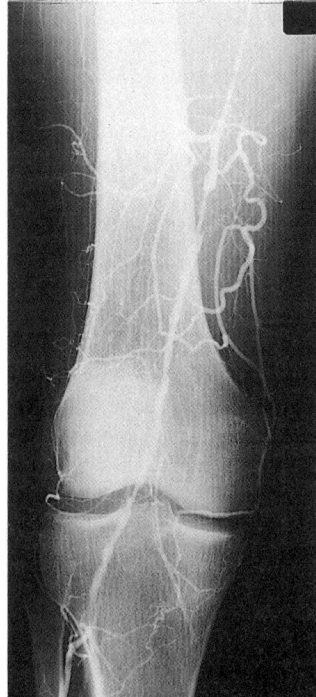

(d)

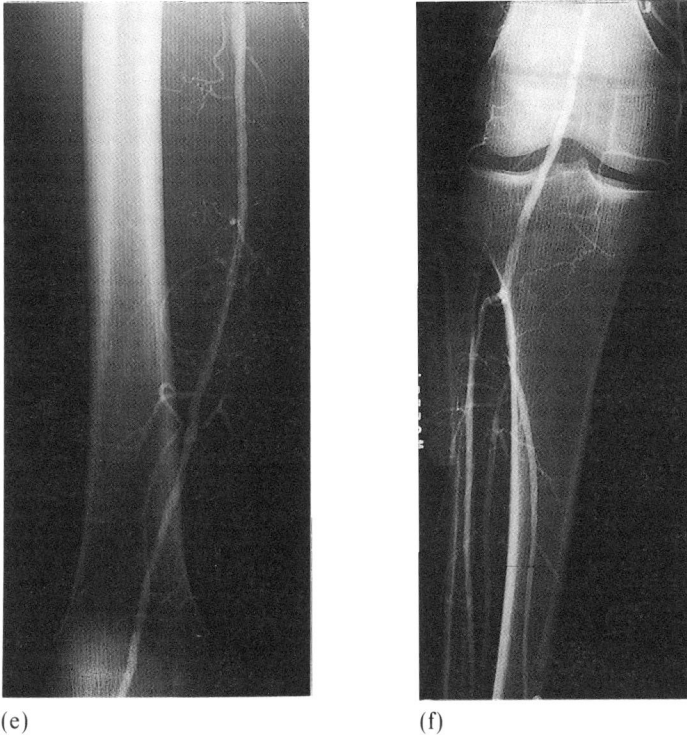

(e)   (f)

Figure 5.11 Pulsed spray thrombolysis. (a) Right superficial femoral artery thrombosis. (b) Extending into popliteal and tibial arteries. (c) Pulsed spray catheter in position across the occlusion with tip occluding guidewire in the thrombus. (d) After successful lysis, multiple stenoses demonstrated. (e), (f) After successful angioplasty

Clinically successful lysis can be achieved in nearly 100% of either native arterial or graft occlusions with a time to lysis of 65 minutes for native arteries and 93 minutes for grafts[30]. Minor complications such as puncture site haematoma and distal embolization occurred in 23% of patients in their subsequent series, in which there was also a major haemorrhagic complication rate of 4%.

The technique of pulsed spray pharmaco-mechanical thrombolysis has also been tried with small pulses of high dose t-PA by Yusuf *et al.*[31] The 5F infusion catheter with multiple side holes, with its end hole occluded by a special tip occluding guidewire, is positioned within the thrombus as above. Each pulse consists of 66 μg of t-PA in 0.2 ml of sterile water, which is injected either forcefully by hand or a specially designed mechanical pump using a 1 ml syringe from a solution containing 0.33 mg/ml every 30 seconds. The pulses of t-PA are delivered until lysis is complete or no longer progressive. The degree of lysis of the thrombus is monitored every 30–60 minutes by repeat arteriography, which may show spasm in the distal vessels. This may be associated with a clinical deterioration in the ischaemic leg and should be treated by the addition of glyceryl trinitrate to the solution. Heparin is not used during pulsed spray thrombolysis, but 3000–5000 units are given before angioplasty if this is required. In a series of 38 patients, clinically successful lysis was achieved in 84% with a median time to lysis of 120 minutes[31].

The problem with the technique is that it is relatively labour intensive, like all accelerated techniques, and the equipment is expensive. Each pulse spray catheter system costs between £150 and £200 and the automatic infusion pump, which is nearing completion of development, will also be expensive (approximately £10 000), although there are cheaper alternatives.

Other techniques of removing thrombus

Distal embolization of small fragments of thrombus complicating either percutaneous transluminal angioplasty or thrombolysis can be treated by thrombolytic infusion over a few hours, or more immediately by the technique of percutaneous aspiration thrombo-embolectomy[32]. This is simply performed by suction of the fragments of fresh thrombus, old thrombus or atheromatous debris into a 6 or 8F gauge catheter, which is then withdrawn through a vascular sheath (Figure 5.12).

Percutaneous aspiration thrombo-embolectomy has been performed successfully in patients with long thrombotic occlusions and has the advantage of achieving arterial patency much faster than thrombolysis alone[33]. The technique often has to be used in combination with angioplasty or thrombolysis.

Catheters with various types of rotating devices at their tips are certainly able to produce fragmentation of thrombus by a mechanical effect in the laboratory and are at present under clinical evaluation[34-36]. Alternatively catheters containing ultrasonic probes can also produce disintegration of thrombus and may become available for clinical use. The potential advantage of mechanical thrombus ablation over drug-induced thrombolysis is that arterial patency could be achieved within a few minutes and this would allow percutaneous treatment of even the most severe acutely ischaemic leg. Distal embolization of micro-fragments of thrombus may be a problem.

The logistics of thrombolysis for the radiologist

Successful thrombolysis requires co-operation between a clinical team consisting of vascular surgeons, radiologists, haematologists, nurses and radiographers. It is, however, a time-consuming method of treating patients with peripheral vascular disease and therefore has significant implications for the department of radiology.

Conventional low-dose infusion thrombolysis certainly has advantages from the radiologist's point of view because the various stages of the procedure (diagnostic arteriography, positioning of the infusion catheter, monitoring arteriography and completion angioplasty) can be arranged at specific suitable times, which are separated by a significant number of hours, when the patient returns to the ward. This technique therefore gives the radiologist some versatility in working practice within the department.

Accelerated methods of thrombolysis, including the pulsed spray technique, have the disadvantage of being very intense in that the radiologist is actively

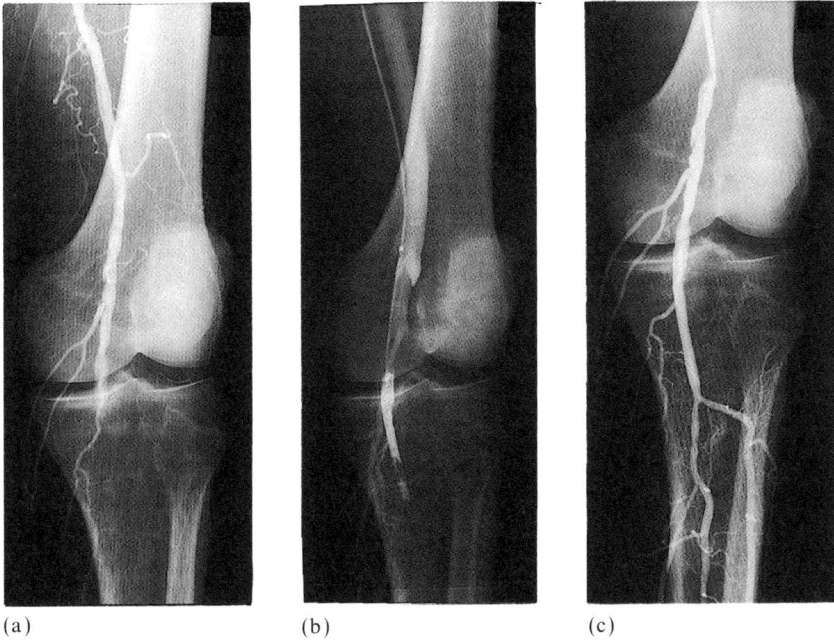

(a)   (b)   (c)

Figure 5.12 Aspiration thrombectomy. (a) Left popliteal artery embolus. (b) Embolus shown distal to angioplasty catheter. (c) After successful catheter aspiration

involved throughout the procedure, which may last as long as 6 hours. These techniques therefore have implications for a busy department, despite their efficiency.

The cost of radiological equipment including pulsed spray and angioplasty catheters used for thrombolysis is not inconsiderable and may add to overstretched departmental budgets. Modern catheter equipment, for example new pulsed spray lysis kits, are individually expensive and often a range of different sizes will need to be stocked. Bulk ordering and local competition may reduce prices but careful evaluation of new equipment is necessary to ensure cost effectiveness. This particularly applies also to the thrombolytic agents themselves. Routine use of t-PA or urokinase can contribute excessively to local radiology budgets.

References

1. van Breda A, Katzen BT and Deutsch AS. Urokinase versus streptokinase in local thrombolysis. *Radiology* 1987; **165**: 109–11
2. Hess H, Mietaschk A and Brückl R. Peripheral arterial occlusions: a 6 year experience with local low-dose thrombolytic therapy. *Radiology* 1987; **163**: 753–8
3. Hess H, Ingrisch H, Mietaschk A and Rath H. Local low-dose thrombolytic therapy of peripheral arterial occlusions. *New Engl J Med* 1982; **307**: 1627–30
4. Earnshaw JJ, Gregson RHS, Makin GS and Hopkinson BR. Early results of low dose intra-arterial streptokinase therapy in acute and subacute lower limb arterial ischaemia. *Br J Surg* 1987; **74**: 504–7

5. Katzen BT and van Breda A. Low dose streptokinase in the treatment of arterial occlusions *AJR* 1981; **136**: 1171–8

6. Allen DR, Faris IB, Ferguson LJ, Miller JH, Lloyd J and Robertson A. Low dose intra-arterial streptokinase in the management of 202 acutely ischaemic legs. *Br J Surg* 1989; **76**: 414

7. Graor RA, Risius B, Young JR, Geisinger MA, Zelch MG, Smith JAM and Ruschhaupt WF. Low-dose streptokinase for selective thrombolysis: systemic effects and complications. *Radiology* 1984; **152**: 35–9

8. Walker WJ and Giddings AEB. A protocol for the safe treatment of acute lower limb ischaemia with intra-arterial streptokinase and surgery. *Br J Surg* 1988; **75**: 1189–92

9. LeBolt SA, Tisnado J, and Cho SR. Treatment of peripheral arterial obstruction with streptokinase; results in arterial versus graft occlusions. *AJR*, 1988; **151**: 589–92

10. Becker GJ, Rabe FE, Richmond BD, Holden RW, Yune HY, Dilley RS, Bang NU, Glover JL and Klatte EC. Low-dose fibrinolytic therapy *Radiology* 1983; **148**: 663–70

11. Belkin M, Belkin B, Bucknam CA, Straub JJ and Lowe R. Intra-arterial fibrinolytic therapy. Efficacy of streptokinase versus urokinase. *Arch Surg* 1986; **121**: 769–73

12. Lammer J, Pilger E, Neumayer K and Schreyer H. Intra-arterial fibrinolysis; long term results. *Radiology* 1986; **161**: 151–63

13. Earnshaw JJ, Westby JC, Gregson RHS, Makin GS and Hopkinson BR. Local thrombolytic therapy of acute peripheral arterial ischaemia with tissue plasminogen activator: a dose-ranging study. *Br J Surg* 1988; **75**: 1196–1200

14. Berridge DC, Gregson RHS, Hopkinson BR and Makin GS. Intra-arterial thrombolysis using recombinant tissue plasminogen activator (r-TPA): the optimal agent, at the optimal dose? *Eur J Vasc Surg* 1989; **3**: 327–32

15. Berridge DC, Gregson RHS, Makin GS and Hopkinson BR. Tissue plasminogen activator in peripheral arterial thrombolysis. *Br J Surg* 1990; **77**: 179–82

16. Earnshaw JJ. Thrombolytic therapy in the management of acute limb ischaemia. *Br J Surg* 1991; **78**: 261–9

17. Berridge DC, Gregson RHS, Hopkinson BR and Makin GS. Randomized trial of intra-arterial recombinant tissue plasminogen activator, intravenous recombinant tissue plasminogen activator and intra-arterial streptokinase in peripheral arterial thrombolysis. *Br J Surg* 1991; **78**: 988–95

18. McNamara TO and Fischer JR. Thrombolysis of peripheral arterial and graft occlusions; improved results using high-dose urokinase. *Am J Roentgenol* 1985; **144**: 769–75

19. McNamara TO. Role of thrombolysis in peripheral arterial occlusion. *Am J Med* 1987; **83** (suppl 2A): 6–10

20. Troughber PD, Cook PS, Micklos TJ and Miller FJ. Intra-arterial fibrinolytic therapy for popliteal and tibial artery obstruction; comparison of streptokinase and urokinase. *Am J Roentgenol* 1987; **149**: 453–6

21. Cragg AH, Smith AP, Corson JD, Nakagawa N, Casteneda E, Kresowik TF, Sharp WJ, Shamma A and Berbaum KS. Two urokinase dose regimens in native arterial and graft occlusions: initial results of a prospective, randomized clinical trial. *Radiology* 1991; **178**: 681–6

22. Verstraete M, Hess H, Mahler, F, Mietaschk, A, Roth FJ, Schneider E, Baert AL and Verhaeghe R. Femoro-popliteal artery thrombolysis with intra-arterial infusion of re-combinant tissue-type plasminogen activator – report of a pilot trial. *Eur J Vasc Surg* 1988; **2**: 155–9

23. Graor RA, Risius B, Lucas FV, Young JR, Ruschhaupt WF, Beven EG and Grossbard EB. Thrombolysis with recombinant human tissue-type plasminogen activator in patients with peripheral and bypass graft occlusions. *Circulation* 1986; **74** (suppl 1): 15–20

24. Risius B, Graor RA, Geisinger MA, Zelch MG, Lucas FV and Young JR. Thrombolytic therapy with recombinant human tissue-type plasminogen activator: a comparison of two doses. *Radiology* 1987; **164**: 465–8

25. Meyerovitz MF, Goldhaber SZ, Reagan K, Polak JF, Kandarpa K, Grassi CJ, Donovan BC, Bettmann MA and Harrington DP. Recombinant tissue-type plasminogen activator

versus urokinase in peripheral arterial and graft occlusions: a randomized trial. *Radiology* 1990; **175**: 75–8

26. Buckenham TM, George CD, Chester JF, Taylor RS and Dormandy JA. Accelerated thrombolysis using pulsed intra-thrombus recombinant human tissue type plasminogen activator (rt-PA). *Eur J Vasc Surg* 1992; **6**: 237–40

27. Braithwaite B, Birch P, Davies C, Poskitt K, Heather BP and Earnshaw JJ. Accelerated high-dose bolus tissue plasminogen activator extends the role of peripheral thrombolysis but may increase risk. *Br J Surg* 1994; **81**: 619

28. Jørgensen B, Tønnesen KH, Bülow J, Nielson JD, Jørgensen M, Holstein P and Anderson E. Femoral artery recanalisation with percutaneous angioplasty and segmentally enclosed plasminogen activator. *Lancet* 1989; **i**: 1106–8

29. Bookstein JJ, Fellmeth B, Roberts A, Valji K, Davis D and Machado T. Pulsed-spray pharmacomechanical thrombolysis: preliminary clinical results. *AJR* 1989; **152**: 1097–1100

30. Valji K, Roberts AC, Davis GB and Bookstein JJ. Pulsed-spray thrombolysis of arterial and bypass graft occlusions. *AJR* 1991; **156**: 617–21

31. Yusuf SW, Whitaker SC, Gregson RHS, Wenham PW, Hopkinson BR, Makin GS. Experience with pulse-spray technique in peripheral thrombolysis. *Eur J Vasc Surg* 1994; **8**: 270–5

32. Belli A-M, Cumberland DC, Knox AM, Procter AE and Welsh CL. The complication rate of percutaneous peripheral balloon angioplasty. *Clin Radiol* 1990; **41**: 380–3

33. Stark EE, McDermott JC, Crummy AB, Turnispeed WD, Acher CW and Burgess JH. Percutaneous aspiration thromboembolectomy. *Radiology* 1985; **156**: 61–6

34. Kensey K, Nash J, Abrahams C and Zarins CK. Recanalization of obstructive arteries with a flexible, rotating tip catheter. *Radiology* 1987; **165**: 387–8

35. Schmitz-Rode T and Günther R. Percutaneous mechanical thrombolysis: a comparative study of various rotational catheter systems. *Invest Radiol* 1991; **26**: 557–63

36. Drasler WJ, Jenson ML, Wilson GJ, Thielen JM, Protonotarios EI, Dutcher RG and Possis ZC. Rheolytic catheter for percutaneous removal of thrombus. *Radiology* 1992; **182**: 263–7

Chapter 6

Graft thrombolysis

T. M. Buckenham

Introduction

The occluded graft poses a complex problem for radiologist and surgeon alike and its successful management relies heavily on the skills and cooperation of both.

There are two aims in graft thrombolysis: to recanalize the run-off vessels and to identify the cause of graft failure facilitating directed percutaneous or surgical management.

Prior to commencing thrombolysis the radiologist should visit the patient on the surgical ward to review the detailed operation notes with a description of the original graft insertion (if available), take a history and examine the affected limb. This review of the clinical situation will enable a planned approach and a better appreciation of the risks and benefits, which should be discussed with the patient.

Essential preliminary information

The following information must be obtained before thrombolysis is attempted.

Type of graft

For the purpose of thrombolysis, grafts can be divided into two groups – prosthetic and non-prosthetic. This is an important distinction as each is managed differently.

Prosthetic grafts are primarily polytetrafluoroethylene (PTFE) or Dacron, which is rarely used below the inguinal ligament. Dacron may be woven or knitted and this is an important distinction as there is a greater risk of extravasation during thrombolysis of the knitted type[1]. Extravasation has also been reported with PTFE[2] and Pulse-Tec[3] grafts (Figure 6.1). Prosthetic grafts are incompressible and maintain their lumen despite chronic occlusion. This facilitates access, for example by direct graft puncture[4,5], and enables easy intra-luminal passage of wires and catheters.

Non-prosthetic grafts are usually saphenous vein, either *in situ* or reversed, but some surgeons use other variations such as human umbilical vein[6]. Vein

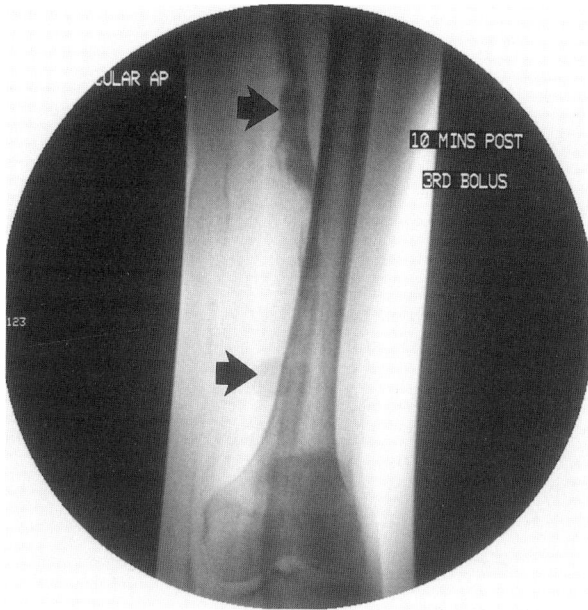

Figure 6.1 Contrast extravasation from a Pulse-Tec graft (arrows)

grafts have a smaller lumen and tend to collapse and fibrose when occluded. They are therefore more difficult to access and can only be reached via a native artery.

Some grafts are a combination of vein and prosthetic material. It is presently believed that the patency of femoro-popliteal PTFE grafts can be enhanced with vein patches and collars[7] (e.g. Taylor Patch or Miller cuff) at the distal anastomosis. Another combination is the composite graft[8] consisting of a prosthetic graft with a distal venous jump graft either used to cross the knee joint or bypass distal anastomotic stenosis.

Anatomy of the graft

The surgical notes should provide information about the location of the anastomoses, ideally using diagrams. Unfortunately in many cases the patient comes from another hospital or the notes are inadequate. This poses a significant problem as it is important to know the location and angle of origin of the graft to facilitate catheterization. The origin may be at an unusual site, such as the external iliac artery, rendering an ipsi-lateral common femoral approach impossible. Metal clips and staples visible on fluoroscopy may provide a clue but can also be misleading. This problem occurs less with prosthetic grafts as they may often be palpated and accessed by direct puncture[4,5].

The operation notes may provide other useful information such as the configuration of the anastomosis, the size of the anastomosed vessel and whether any interposing material has been used to form a patch or cuff. The presence of a jump graft, or even a second graft, is important when considering percutaneous intervention at the end of thrombolysis. Some patients have had multiple grafts inserted on different occasions. The presence of an older thrombosed graft is particularly important as it may be very difficult to decide radiologically which is the recently occluded graft and hence the one to treat with thrombolysis.

Duration of occlusion

It is often difficult to decide how long a graft has been occluded. Many patients do not give a history of a sudden event resulting in deterioration of symptoms. Review of serial ankle brachial indices may show a sudden drop in pressure suggesting a graft occlusion. Careful questioning of the patient usually gives an indication of the duration of clinical deterioration and for practical purposes this can be taken as the time of occlusion.

Grafts with a recent occlusion are easier to lyse but conversely old occlusions are not always impossible to treat. A history of less than 6 months would be sufficient indication to attempt a trial of thrombolysis but the radiologist should be prepared to stop if no progress is made.

Physical examination

Careful palpation of pulses is important to assess the possible points of access to the vascular tree. For example, if a patient with an aorto-bifemoral graft has no femoral pulses this limits access sites to the arm or direct graft puncture[4] under ultrasound control. The procedure is technically more difficult and, if the arm is used, potentially more hazardous[9].

Infra-inguinal prosthetic grafts are often easy to palpate which enables the radiologist to determine their origin and insertion and a site of possible graft puncture. If more than one thrombosed graft is palpable it is impossible to determine on physical examination which of them is more recently occluded. In these cases puncture of the graft and examination of the aspirated material is useful. The fluid is brown and thick or serous if the graft occlusion is very old.

Imaging and accessing the grafts

Angiography is important and will help in selection of an appropriate access point for thrombolysis. Intravenous digital subtraction angiography (IV DSA) is very useful as it provides adequate images without requiring an arterial puncture. IV DSA will often define the patency of the run-off vessels. If these are patent the lysis procedure has a better prognosis and this correlates with less severe ischaemia clinically. Non-filling of the distal vessels on IV DSA does not necessarily imply their occlusion as distal opacification may be poor in the face of proximal occlusion[10].

Once the angiogram has demonstrated the occluded graft and the patent distal vessels, the site of access may be chosen. Once access has been secured, insertion of a sheath is useful. It allows rapid painless catheter exchange, repeated angiography and drug adminstration. A sheath with a detachable hub is an advantage if aspiration thrombectomy is considered.

Femoro-popliteal grafts

Femoro-popliteal vein grafts may be approached from the contralateral groin and a wire passed over the bifurcation with the use of a Simmons or Cobra type catheter. Accessing the graft origin can be difficult and is best achieved with these catheters and an angled hydrophilic guidewire. Most vein grafts arise antero-medially from the common femoral artery. If the wire can be directed by the catheter it will 'run' along the expected medial line of the graft, but getting the catheter to follow may be difficult and exchange to a stiffer wire may be necessary. The ipsi-lateral common femoral artery may be accessed but this is very difficult in the obese patient as the puncture site may be below the origin of the graft. Even if the puncture is proximal to the graft origin there is often very little distance between the two, making catheter manipulation difficult. In this situation the wire may be passed into the superficial femoral or profunda femoris arteries and a dilator passed over it. The dilator is then replaced by an angled Berenstein catheter and withdrawn whilst injecting contrast until the tip is only just lying in the common femoral artery. The angled tip can then be used to direct the wire into the graft. A high puncture in the external iliac artery may be tempting in these cases but is contra-indicated when thrombolytic agent is given due to the risk of retroperitoneal bleeding.

Femoro-popliteal prosthetic grafts may also be accessed using the same techniques but the same difficulties arise. Scar tissue in the ipsi-lateral groin, which is more marked with prosthetic grafts, makes an ipsilateral common femoral artery approach even more difficult. There are, however, advantages of this approach, if it can be achieved. There is a direct line of access to the distal anastomosis and run-off vessels allowing angioplasty or atherectomy and also enabling aspiration thrombectomy to be performed.

A useful option with prosthetic grafts is accessing the lumen by direct puncture of the anterior wall of the graft in the most proximal palpable site[4]. This allows rapid access for aspiration thrombectomy and thrombolysis. This technique involves locating the graft with ultrasound or by palpation and puncturing the anterior wall only with a single piece needle. Once the needle tip is in the lumen the guidewire will run freely down the graft and a sheath may be inserted. Limitations of this technique are the difficulty of only puncturing the anterior wall and the inability to image the proximal anastomosis after lysis. It should be remembered that this technique requires prophylactic antibiotics.

Aorto-bifemoral grafts

Thrombolysis of retroperitoneal aorto-iliac and aorto-bifemoral grafts requires caution because of the possibility of uncontrollable haemorrhage through the interstices of the graft. This situation may be a specific indication for aspiration thrombectomy instead of thrombolysis (see later). If it is decided to use lysis, extreme vigilance must be exercised. If one limb of an aorto-bifemoral graft is occluded catheter access can usually be obtained via

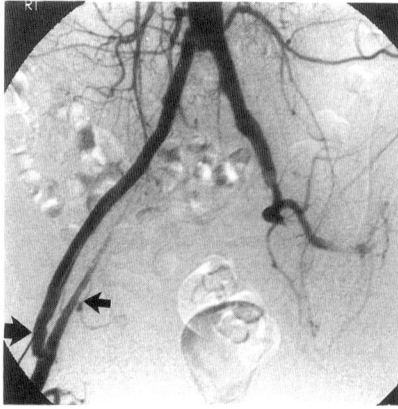

(a)

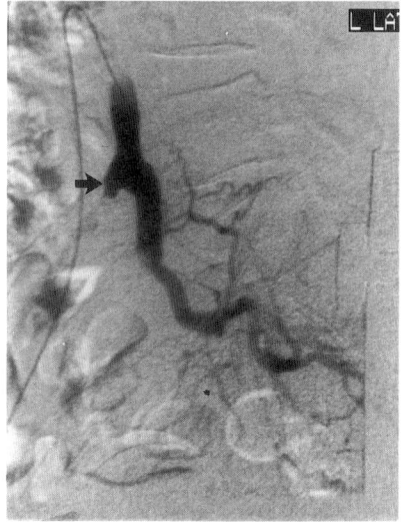

(b)

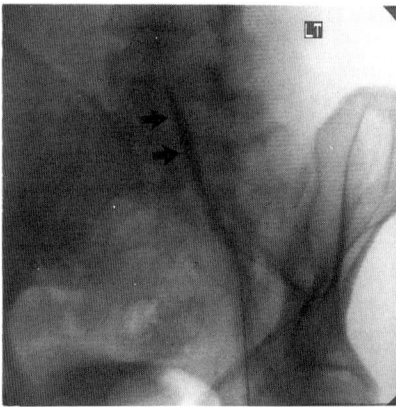

(c)

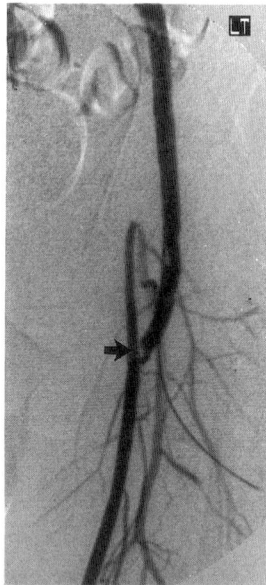

(d)

the contralateral groin. If both limbs of the graft are occluded, the alternatives are the axillary/brachial route or direct puncture of the occluded graft in the groin. This latter method of accessing grafts 'downstream' from the proximal point of occlusion, whilst unconventional, is highly effective in this and other situations where a proximal graft is occluded in the groin (Figure 6.2). The catheter tip should be placed near the proximal end of the occlusion for infusion. The incidence of puncture site haemorrhage is no higher than with conventional techniques.

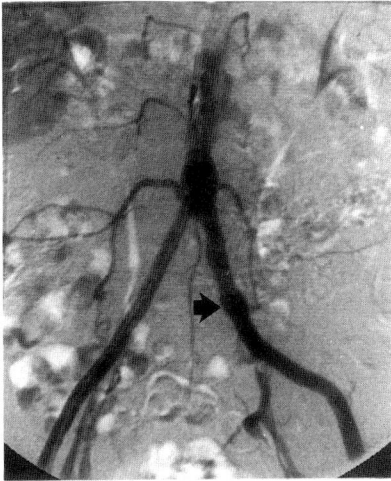

(e)

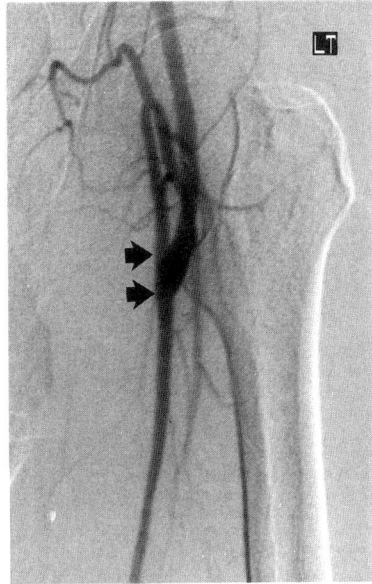

(f)

Figure 6.2 (a) A 65-year-old man with bilateral ilio-femoral Dacron grafts. Acute occlusion on the left side, angiogram has been performed via the patent right graft (arrow). Note native iliac artery back filling (small arrow). (b) The origin of the left ilio-femoral graft could not be identified for access despite imaging in the lateral projection. Note the occluded external iliac artery (arrow). (c) Direct puncture of the occluded left ilio-femoral graft (arrows) in the ipsilateral groin has permitted successful thrombolysis and balloon dilatation of the proximal iliac artery. (d) Neointimal hyperplasia of the distal anastomosis (arrow). The distal anastomosis was revised with a vein patch. (e), (f) Angiogram 6 months later showing patent graft with widely open proximal and distal anastomoses (arrows)

Extra-anatomic grafts

Grafts such as axillo-bifemoral and femoro-femoral cross-over grafts are very difficult to access by conventional means. The cross-over graft has to be approached from the donor common femoral artery and a wire manipulated into the graft origin. This is often impossible and direct puncture may be the only option[5]. Axillo-bifemoral grafts may be approached via the axillary artery route, but this limits catheter manipulation and the catheter has to remain across the origin of the vertebral artery with the risk of embolization. Direct graft puncture over the chest wall or preferably in either groin are options in these difficult grafts.

Aspiration thrombectomy

Once the sheath is inserted via an ipsi-lateral puncture it is often possible to debulk the graft thrombus by using aspiration. This is particularly the case in prosthetic grafts as the lumen is maintained despite occlusion. A large bore 7F (0.074 in) non-tapered catheter is passed to the level of the distal anastomosis and aspiration carried out by hand using a 50 ml syringe as the catheter is withdrawn. Often the thrombus lodges in the sheath, hence the

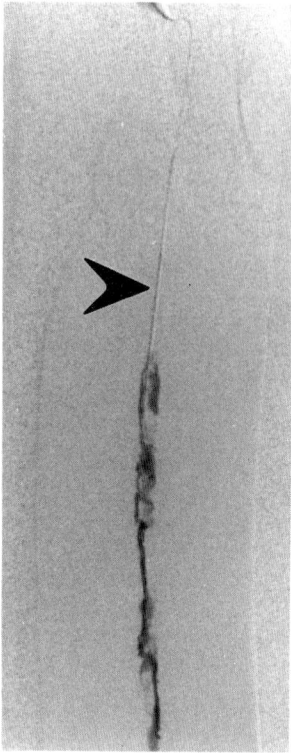

(a)

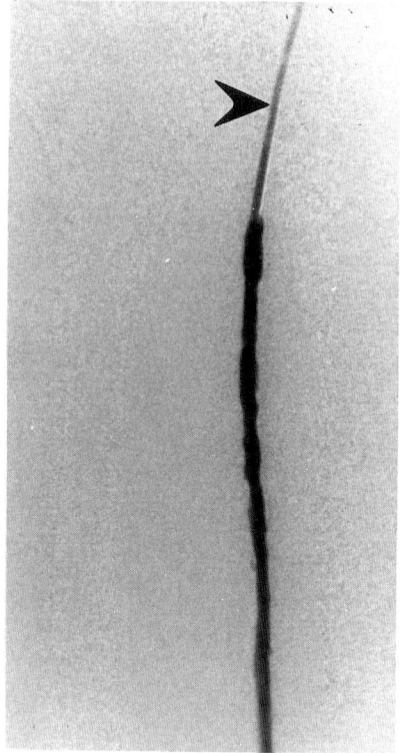

(b)

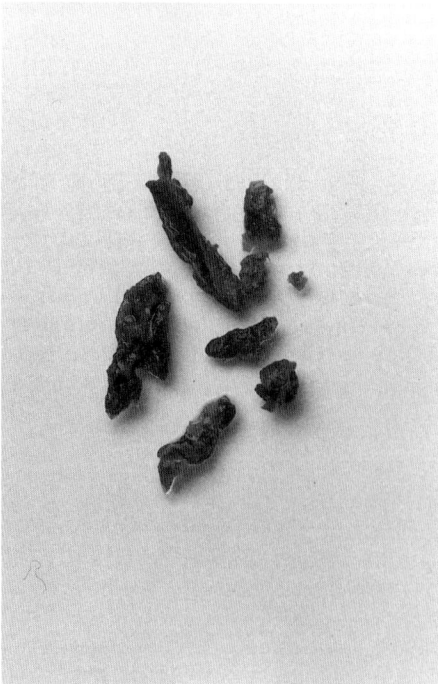

(c)

Figure 6.3 Aspiration thrombectomy of superficial femoral artery thrombosis. (a) Thrombus clearly visible in superficial femoral artery. Access sheath arrowed. (b) After aspiration thrombectomy. Aspiration catheter arrowed. (c) Fragments of aspirated thrombus

need for a removable hub allowing the clot to be withdrawn. It is difficult to be precise about the correct time to embark on aspiration. Often, at the commencement of the procedure, clot is difficult to aspirate but after initial administration of thrombolytic agent the thrombus becomes softer and easier to aspirate. The age of the thrombus is an important consideration as fresh clots are easier to aspirate. It often becomes a matter of 'suck it and see'.

There are more sophisticated aspiration devices currently available; most work on the principle of emulsifying the clot prior to its removal. This may be effected by using a wire or a high-pressure jet of saline. These catheters are, as yet, far from perfect but are rapidly developing and may become a useful treatment option.

The disadvantage of aspiration is that a large puncture site (7–8F) is needed which increases the risk of haemorrhage. The risk of distal embolization is unknown. Due to the smooth wall of a graft, aspiration catheters are less likely to cause intimal damage than in a native artery and do not need to be placed over a guide wire as long as they are confined to the graft itself.

Generally, repeated aspiration of the graft with a non-tapering 7F catheter will accelerate lysis and help to remove any insoluble component such as an embolus lying within the graft. The run-off vessels may also be aspirated but this has to be performed with a tapered 5F catheter introduced over a guide wire and is more hazardous (Figure 6.3).

Thrombolysis

There are many infusion regimens for delivering thrombolytic agents but there are some specific features of graft thrombolysis that are worth emphasising. Unlike a native vessel a thrombosed graft has no side branches and often one end is partially closed (usually a stenosed distal anastomosis). If a large volume of lytic agent is injected directly into the graft, thrombus can accidentally be displaced distally into the run-off vessels or proximally into the common femoral or profunda femoris arteries (whirlpool effect). To prevent this occurring, the clot may be debulked with a suction catheter and the lytic agent injected slowly throughout the length of the graft. For the same reason it is preferable to give multiple small aliquots than larger bolus doses. The regimen we use is 5 mg t-PA given as a bolus up to a maximum dose of 15 mg[11,12]. The high-dose boluses may be followed by an infusion of 0.05 mg/kg/h t-PA if needed for up to 4 hours. It may be prudent to place a distal occluding balloon in those cases where the run off is patent and not protected by a distal anastomotic stenosis. Alternatively, graft thrombolysis may be performed using standard low-dose infusion techniques with t-PA or streptokinase.

In cases where the run off is also thrombosed a hydrophilic guidewire can be passed through a distal anastomosis followed by a 3F straight catheter and lytic agent introduced directly into the tibial vessels.

Maintaining patency

Once flow has been established the radiologist is confronted with the most difficult aspect of graft thrombolysis: identifying the cause of graft failure

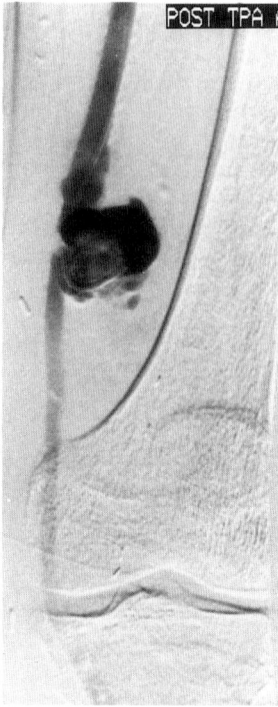

(a)

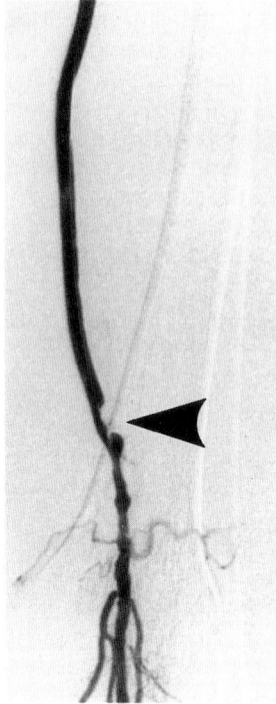

(b)

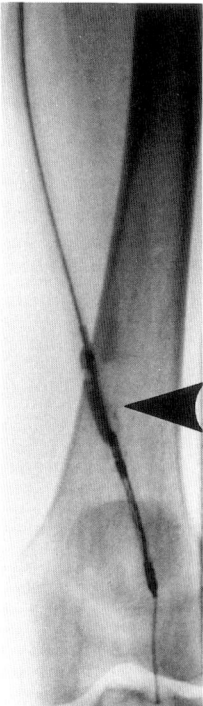

(c)

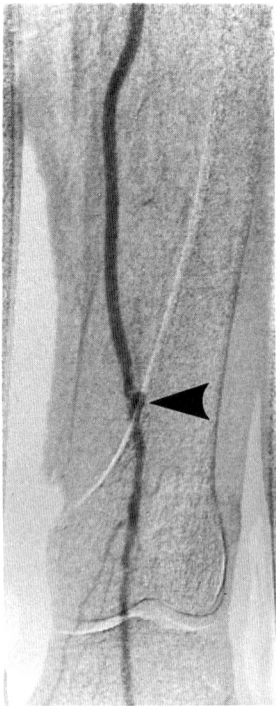

(d)

Figure 6.4 Causes of graft failure.
(a) Infected anastomotic pseudoaneurysm.
(b)–(d) Anastomotic neointimal hyperplasia: management with atherectomy.
(b) Neointimal hyperplasia at distal anastomosis (arrow).
(c) Simpson atherectomy catheter *in situ* (arrow).
(d) Angiographic appearance after percutaneous removal of intimal hyperplasia (anastomosis arrowed)

(Figure 6.4(a)). Grafts fail for three reasons; an inflow problem, an outflow problem or a lesion inherent to the graft itself. Early occlusion of a graft suggests an intrinsic abnormality of the graft or failure to recognize a technical problem on the per-operative angiogram.

Late occlusion is frequently due to inflow or outflow problems which arise as the result of anastomotic neointimal hyperplasia or progression of proximal or distal disease[13,14].

The distal anastomosis is much more commonly affected than the proximal, and significant progression of disease is usually seen in the popliteal or tibial vessels rather than in the aorta or iliac arteries. Careful imaging is mandatory to ascertain the cause of failure, enabling early treatment by endovascular techniques or surgery. Angiography of the anastomosis should be performed in two planes, and if the distal anastomosis is in the distal popliteal artery or below, a flexed knee lateral view should be included. The run-off vessels should be clearly imaged as far as the feet and any suspicious lesions viewed in the oblique plane.

Typical patterns of disease are often seen which give good indications for subsequent management. For instance, anastomotic neointimal hyperplasia appears as a single discrete filling defect 1–2 cm proximal to the distal anastomosis at the heel of the graft. Balloon dilatation is not usually effective in treating neointimal hyperplasia and the patient requires surgical management. If surgery is contra-indicated for any reason, an atherectomy catheter may be used to remove the anastomotic hyperplasia, although the long-term efficacy of this technique is unknown (Figure 6.4(b)–(d)).

Progression of atheromatous disease within native vessels can usually be managed with balloon angioplasty[15] and, if experienced, there should be no hesitation in dilating significant infra-popliteal stenoses.[16]

Rarely the lesion will lie within the graft itself. Vein grafts may develop strictures as a result of per-operative trauma and these are readily dilated with a conventional angioplasty balloon[17] if less than 1 cm in length. Longer stenoses are best treated by graft revision or patch angioplasty.

Results

Graft thrombolysis has gained popularity due to the poor results of graft thrombectomy. Three-year patency for thrombectomy of below-knee femoro-popliteal prosthetic grafts is as low as 16%[18]. Re-operation of femoro-popliteal prosthetic grafts to isolated popliteal segments yielded annual patency rates even lower (8%)[13]. Graft revision, e.g. patch angioplasty, graft extension or replacement rather than thrombectomy has an improved patency of up to 52% at 3 years for femoro-popliteal grafts and 15% for femoro-tibial grafts[13], but this surgery becomes technically increasingly difficult due to scar tissue and lack of autogenous vein.

Graft recanalization using thrombolysis allows accurate identification of the cause of occlusion and enables more logical management either by angioplasty or surgery (or amputation) with possible advantage in long-term patency, particularly if saphenous vein is not available for reconstruction.

It is difficult to determine medium or long-term patency for grafts treated with thrombolysis. Most reported series only include grafts that could be accessed (cross-over grafts are often excluded) and exclude those patients with severe ischaemia. The reported results of graft lysis are often mixed with those of native vessels.

Of those series which included all types of grafts, the expected patency rate at 1 year was 40–60%. Correction of flow limiting lesions has a dramatic effect on results, improving patency to as much as 88% at 1 year[19].

In our own series of 23 patients with 30 graft occlusions treated with pulsed high-dose t-PA, the average duration of lysis was $2\frac{1}{2}$ hours[20]. Although 72% had patency maintained after thrombolysis, only 48% were patent at 6 months despite correction of the underlying cause by angioplasty or surgery where possible. This series, however, included patients whose grafts had been thrombosed for up to 6 months. Complications were infrequent and appeared to be least for patients in whom the thrombosed graft was accessed by direct puncture. Best results were obtained for occluded femoro-femoral cross-over grafts.

Conclusion

In the absence of autogenous vein for graft revision, thrombolysis is the preferred initial intervention for graft thrombosis. Even when vein is available it is a useful initial option. At least half the patients with successful graft thrombolysis require surgical correction of the causative lesion if long-term patency is to be anticipated. Therefore graft thrombolysis should be undertaken only cautiously in patients not fit for revisional surgery. Some will, however, benefit from thrombolysis combined with angioplasty or anticoagulation.

Perhaps the most important aspect of graft thrombolysis is understanding that clot lysis is often not in itself a treatment, but a diagnostic method with which to uncover the cause of occlusion, re-establish run-off patency and enable more appropriate intervention to establish prolonged patency. It can be concluded that thrombolysis and surgery are not competing alternatives for graft occlusion but are best used selectively, and often in combination.

References

1. Rabe FE, Becker GJ, Richmond BD, Yune HY, Holden RW, Dilley RS and Klatte EC. Contrast extravasation through Dacron grafts: a sequela of low-dose streptokinase therapy. *AJR* 1982; **138**: 917–20
2. Becker GJ, Holden RW and Rabe FE. Contrast extravasation from a Gore-Tex graft: a complication of thrombolytic therapy. *AJR* 1984; **42**: 573–4
3. Buckenham TM, Taylor RS, Reiff D and Page JE. Contrast extravasation from a Pulse-Tec graft: a complication of high-dose recombinant tissue-type plasminogen activator therapy. *Br J Radiol* 1992; **65**: 545–7
4. Page JE, Buckenham TM and Taylor RS. Accelerated thrombolysis facilitated by direct puncture of occluded prosthetic femoral grafts. *Australas. Radiol.* 1992; **36**: 230–3
5. Buckenham TM, George CD, Taylor RS and Dormandy JA. Thrombolysis and the femorofemoral bypass graft: a new technique. *Australas Radiol* 1992; **36**: 99–101
6. Dardik H, Ibrahim IM and Dardik JD. Femoral tibial-peroneal bypass. The lateral approach and the use of glutaraldehyde tanned umbilical vein. *Am J Surg* 1977; **134**: 199–201
7. Taylor RS, Loh A, McFarland RJ, Cox M and Chester JF. Improved technique for

polytetrafluoroethylene bypass grafting: long-term results using anastomotic vein patches. *Br J Surg* 1992; **79**: 348–54

8. Gregory RT, Raithel D, Snyder SO, Wheeler JR and Gayle RG. Composite grafts: an alternative to saphenous vein for lower extremity arterial reconstruction. *J Cardiovasc Surg.* 1983; **24**: 53–7

9. Hessel SJ, Adams DF and Abrams HL. Complications of angiography. *Radiology* 1981; **138**: 273

10. Van Breda A. Technique of digital subtraction angiography. In: Van Breda A, Katzen BT (eds) *Digital Subtraction Angiography: Practical Aspects.* Slack, Thrace, New Jersey

11. Juhan C, Haupert S, Miltgen G and Barthelemy P. Intra-arterial infusion of rTPA. A two stage procedure. *J Cardiovasc Surg* 1990; **31**: 89

12. Buckenham TM, George CD, Chester JF, Taylor RS and Dormandy JA. Accelerated thrombolysis using pulsed intra-thrombus recombinant human tissue type plasminogen activator (rt-PA). *Eur J Vasc Surg* 1992; **6**: 237–40

13. Ascer E, Collier P, Gupta SK and Veith FJ. Reoperation for PTFE bypass failure: the importance of distal outflow site and operative technique in determining outcome. *J Vasc Surg* 1987; **5**: 298–308

14. Clowes AW and Reidy MA. Prevention of stenosis after vascular reconstruction: pharmacologic control of intimal hyperplasia – a review. *J Vasc Surg* 1991; **13**: 885–91

15. Gardiner G, Harrington D, Koltun W, Whittemore A, Mannick J and Levin D. Salvage of occluded arterial bypass grafts by means of thrombolysis. *J Vasc Surg* 1989; **9**: 426–31

16. Buckenham TM, Aoh A, Dormandy JA and Taylor RS. Infrapopliteal angioplasty for limb salvage. *Eur J Vasc Surg* 1993; **7**: 21–5

17. Sniderman KW, Kalman PG, Shewchun and Goldberg RE. Lower extremities *in situ* saphenous vein grafts. Angiographic interventions. *Radiology* 1989; **170**: 1023–7

18. Whittemore AD, Clowes AW, Couch NP and Mannick JA. Secondary femoropopliteal reconstruction. *Ann Surg* 1981; **193**: 35–42

19. Sullivan K, Gardner G, Kandarpa K *et al.* Efficacy of thrombolysis in infrainguinal bypass grafts. *Circulation* 1991; **83** (suppl I): 99–105

20. Guest P and Buckenham T. Thrombolysis of the occluded prosthetic graft with tissue-type plasminogen activator, results and problems in 23 patients. *Clin Radiol* 1992; **46**: 381–6

Chapter 7

Avoiding the complications of thrombolysis

K. J. Dawson and G. Hamilton

Introduction

Whilst cost and technical complexity may discourage clinicians from undertaking a thrombolytic programme, perhaps the fear of major complications is a more significant factor in reluctance to implement this method. Clearly, attention to reducing complications must be an important feature of any thrombolysis programme. Many different factors can lead to complications. Obviously, correct patient selection is vital, as is expert evaluation of the degree of limb ischaemia and its viability. Individual patients differ markedly in risk factors for a bleeding diathesis. Correct thrombolytic technique, agents and equipment are also important. Monitoring of patients, the level of nursing care and the ward setting are also influential considerations in keeping complications to a minimum. Specific complications to consider and avoid are listed in Table 7.1.

All units with established thrombolytic programmes have negotiated a learning curve to reach a point where the balance of risk and benefit is weighted in favour of treating an individual patient with thrombolysis. Clinicians wishing to begin using thrombolysis will want to learn from the lessons of others and achieve good clinical results with a minimum of

Table 7.1 Complications of thrombolysis

A. Bleeding
   Puncture site bleeding
   Groin haematoma
   Cerebrovascular accident
   Retroperitoneal haemorrhage
   Muscle haematoma
   Other haemorrhage

B. Pericatheter thrombus

C. Reperfusion syndrome

D. Distal embolization

E. Allergic reactions

F. Arterial/graft perforation

G. Catheter-related problems

morbidity and mortality. A few complications will undoubtedly occur despite the best precautions. However, many are preventable and can be avoided by strict attention to detail.

Patient selection

The initial clinical evaluation is critical in ensuring that the appropriate patients undergo treatment[1]. A paralysed, paraesthetic limb with skin mottling and muscle tenderness is clearly beyond salvage, and restoration of blood flow, however briefly, will cause a reperfusion syndrome with a high probability of death. Clearly thrombolysis is not to be considered in such a case. At the other end of the spectrum is a patient presenting with a short (several hours) history of rest pain due to an occluded prosthetic peripheral bypass graft in a limb that is clinically viable. Treatment of this patient with thrombolysis is very likely to restore graft blood flow and return this limb to normal in a short period. Between these extremes is a spectrum of clinical presentations and circumstances. It is of paramount importance that evaluation should be undertaken by a vascular specialist experienced in dealing with limb ischaemia so that appropriate treatment can be instigated rapidly.

Indications for intra-arterial thrombolysis (Table 7.2) have been discussed in detail elsewhere[1], as have contra-indications. Certain points need emphasis in the context of avoiding complications.

Patients with a bleeding diathesis should be excluded and therefore those who are within weeks of intra-cranial, intra-abdominal or intra-thoracic surgery should not undergo thrombolysis. There is little in the literature to guide us in this regard and conventionally 6 weeks is taken as the danger period following surgery, though the type of surgery undertaken may be more relevant than the duration since operation. Intra-abdominal or intra-thoracic procedures that leave large raw surfaces, e.g. lung decortication, splenectomy, partial hepatectomy, will be more risky than procedures which cause less disruption of tissue. Small bleeds within the skull will have major consequences and therefore extreme care should be taken following neuro-surgery. The danger period of about 6 weeks may have to be extended in high-risk cases.

Table 7.2 Indications for intra-arterial thrombolysis

Well established	Less well established
Acute limb ischaemia	Stroke
Vascular graft occlusion	Limb small vessel occlusion
Neglected arterial emboli	Acute mesenteric ischaemia
Thrombosed popliteal aneurysms	Dural venous sinus thrombosis
Vascular access device occlusion	Hepatic venous occlusion
Major vein thrombosis	
Visceral arterial thrombosis	

Patients with a history of peptic ulceration or recurrent dyspepsia should probably have gastroscopy before embarking on treatment, as re-activation of a bleeding peptic ulcer may occur and haemorrhage can be severe. If there is no time available for gastroscopy, prophylactic treatment with anti-ulcer drugs is an alternative. An antecedent history of haemorrhagic stroke is a contra-indication to thrombolysis. Great care should be taken with patients who are taking oral anticoagulants. Warfarin therapy should be changed to heparin infusion which is easier to monitor and reverse.

Bleeding will occur through arteriotomy suture lines and therefore thrombolysis should be rarely and very carefully undertaken if arterial surgery, e.g. embolectomy, has been done recently. If necessary, infusion of a thrombolytic drug should be below any suture lines and great care must be taken with positioning of the catheter. If a combination of thrombolysis and surgery is considered, it is best to use thrombolysis first, not only to restore patency but as a means of improving the chances of reconstruction by clearing run-off vessels. Agents with a short half-life can be used right up to the time of anaesthetic induction if surgery is required. Thus intra-arterial thrombolysis can act as a diagnostic aid in addition to its therapeutic advantages.

Demented, disturbed or uncooperative patients who will not remain still or lie flat and who may interfere with or dislodge intra-arterial catheters should be treated by other means if possible. These are the situations in which catheter-related problems such as kinking and breakage are common. Movement of the catheter and pressure on the arterial wall if the treated limb is repeatedly flexed can cause vessel perforation at the site of impaction of the catheter tip.

Technique

Having decided that thrombolysis is the right method of treatment then it is important to ensure that the correct radiological technique is used. There are many variations of technique and these have been discussed in detail in other chapters. Certain points, however, require emphasis if complications are to be avoided.

A contra-lateral common femoral artery puncture is generally used[2]. This ensures that the puncture site is not exposed to the thrombolytic infusion, thus minimizing puncture site bleeding.

The common femoral artery is the preferred puncture site as it is easily accessible and can be readily compressed. Access via arm vessels is technically more difficult and may be less satisfactory due to the incidence of vessel spasm and difficulty in controlling bleeding after catheter removal. The trans-lumbar, aortic route is unsuitable as puncture site bleeding here is uncontrollable. In our experience, the use of a catheter introducer sheath (Figure 7.1) has been invaluable in minimizing both patient pain and vessel trauma during repeat catheter manipulations and check angiography[2,3]. All subsequent check studies, catheter changes and angioplasties are performed via this sheath. Thus the vessel is only punctured once. The sheath side arm is perfused with either a small dose of thrombolytic drug or a heparin solution.

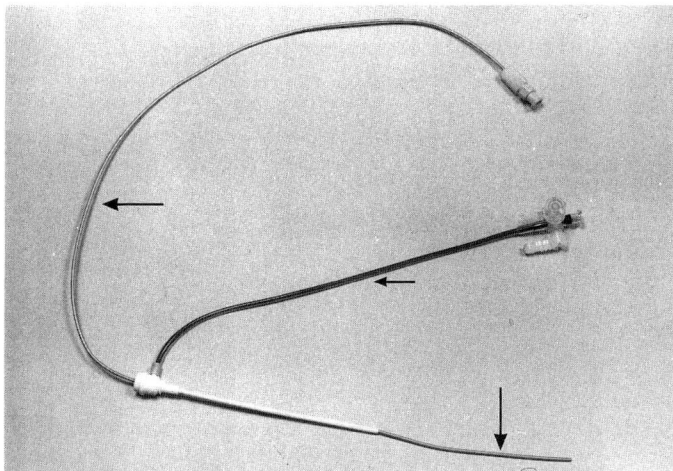

Figure 7.1 Catheter introducer sheath. Large arrows = infusion catheter; small arrow = sheath side arm

The thrombolytic agent is made up in solution with normal saline and infused in a volume of about 10 ml per hour. Smaller volumes tend to be lost in catheter dead space. A standard infusion pump is used and it is essential to ensure not only that the pump works correctly but that its function during infusion is maintained. This requires prompt attention from trained staff in the event of pump alarms indicating a problem. Should there be a problem with the infusion, arterial pressure will force blood back into the infusion tube, which will rapidly clot. Dislodging this thrombus by flushing will merely fill the treated vessel with further thrombotic material.

To prevent catheter thrombosis during transit between the radiology department and the ward, the infusion should be set up and started in the angiography suite, and a battery-driven pump is essential.

Simple but effective methods to secure the catheter should be used to prevent it being dislodged. Inadvertent removal of an intra-arterial catheter is potentially catastrophic if the haemorrhage is unnoticed. This is particularly a problem in patients who become confused, and a fairly common problem in elderly patients treated with streptokinase. The benefit of a catheter introducer sheath can be noted in this situation, where if the catheter is accidentally withdrawn, the haemostatic valve will prevent major haemorrhage. It is our policy to fix the catheter and infusion lines firmly to the skin with Tegaderm, a clear plastic adhesive. Other catheter-related problems may occur if the patient is restless or the catheter not adequately secured. The catheter tip may migrate, e.g. from the engaged origin of an occluded femoro-popliteal graft into the profunda femoris orifice. This will siphon thrombolytic drug away from the desired site of action. Movement of the catheter tip within a mobile segment of artery, e.g. the popliteal segment, may cause vessel perforation or promote a subsequent stenosis.

The introduction of infection through an infusion, particularly one taking place over several days, is a real danger and catheter entry through an area of infected skin should be avoided. It is important that all catheters are introduced using full aseptic technique and that there is a closed system for infusion. A catheter left in an unsterile state outside the patient should not be advanced further into the arterial system. It is preferable to have frequent catheter exchanges during thrombolysis, keeping the catheter enclosed within a sterile barrier, rather than run the risk of avoidable infection. Infection at the catheter site is rare but particular care should be taken when a prosthetic graft has been punctured directly. On these occasions it is advisable to give systemic antibiotic prophylaxis.

Nursing care

Patients should be nursed flat to prevent catheter problems such as kinking or breakage, migration and perforation. Observations are made as for a post-operative patient, i.e. 15–30 minute observations of blood pressure, pulse and puncture sites. In the legs, observations are made of skin temperature and colour, sensory and motor function and the presence or absence of calf muscle tenderness noted. We have adopted the nursing care plan format to design a simple instruction chart for ward staff to follow in the nursing care of these patients (Figure 7.2). This is kept with the standard nursing care plan. The familiar format ensures that non-qualified or new staff, unfamiliar with these patients' particular needs, can be guided as to the observations required. Some teams monitor patients on the intensive care unit, but this level of nursing is not necessary and patients can routinely be monitored on vascular surgical wards.

There is undoubtedly a learning curve of experience with both junior medical staff and nurses with regard to management of intra-arterial thrombolytic infusions. It is imperative that fixed protocols be drawn up by senior personnel and displayed prominently in the relevant wards. These should be shown to successive changes of junior medical staff and shift changes of nurses. Only in this way will the correct dilutions and infusion regimens be used and complications due to overdose avoided. It is particularly important to ensure that, unlike intravenous therapy, infusion bags are never allowed to run through as this will cause back bleeding into the giving set and thrombosis of the infusion lines. Most infusions are delivered via infusion pumps which will alarm when the infusion is about to run out. The next infusion bag should be ready for immediate connection. Many of these problems will occur out of hours and it is essential that night nursing staff are familiar with these procedures. Thrombolysis patients should preferably be nursed on one designated ward where the staff are trained to avoid these problems. In our experience a lot of effort was needed to ensure that all staff are capable of managing these infusions around the clock. The input of an interested senior nurse is invaluable. We have used a dedicated thrombolysis staff nurse/sister whose duty it is to liaise between surgical, radiology and nursing staff to ensure smooth running of the thrombolysis service. This individual is uniquely placed to understand the difficulties and priorities of the various staff involved in a thrombolysis programme and to introduce systems to avoid problems. The education of nursing and junior medical

NURSING CARE PLAN FOR PATIENT RECEIVING THROMBOLYTIC THERAPY

	PROBLEM/NEED	AIM	NURSING ACTIONS/INVOLVEMENT
1.	RISK OF HAEMORRHAGE	DETECT EARLY SIGNS	1. Hourly pulse and blood pressure 2. Report tachycardia 3. Report hypotension 4. Observe arterial catheter site for bleeding, bruising and haematoma and report immediately 5. Mark extent of haematoma on skin and document fully in the Nursing Notes 6. Observe any pre-existing haemostatic thrombus sites such as previous arterial puncture sites 7. Check correct dose of thrombolytic agent is being delivered 8. Flat bed rest 9. Ensure patient receives high dependency care
2.	DISCOMFORT/PAIN	MINIMIZE	1. Identify location, type, degree of pain 2. Assess condition of limb 3. Administer adequate analgesia as prescribed 4. Evaluate effect 5. Adequate explanation of situation 6. Spenco mattress or similar pressure relief device 7. Call bell and belongings close at hand
3.	RISK OF DISLODGING THE ARTERIAL CATHETER	MAINTAIN THE CATHETER IN THE CORRECT POSITION	1. Ensure the arterial catheter is held firmly in place with clear adhesive dressing such as Tegaderm 2. Flat bed rest 3. Ensure patient understands the need to lie flat 4. The head of the bed not to be elevated to more than a forty degree angle
4.	RISK OF THE ARTERIAL CATHETER BECOMING THROMBOSED	PREVENT THE CATHETER FROM THROMBOSING	1. Never allow the infusion to stop 2. Prepare a fresh infusion in advance 3. Check all taps are open and the lines are patent 4. Check the dose rate is correct 5. Check the infusion pump is operating correctly 6. Check the condition of the limb 7. Check colour, temperature, sensitivity, ability to move the toes and for any pulses present 8. Report any changes immediately

Figure 7.2 Nursing care plan

staff, supervision and setting up of infusions, and designing of care plans are all within the scope of this individual's duties. Although not absolutely necessary to establish a service, we have found a dedicated thrombolysis nurse to be of such benefit that we would strongly recommend this policy wherever possible. No changes should be made to the infusion or catheters without prior discussion with the vascular specialist. Clear marking of all infusion lines, tubes and infusion bags with labels should be routine.

Repeat angiography, catheter manipulation and vessel compression after thrombolysis are all painful. There is also a certain amount of apprehension as patients understand the threat to their limb. Therefore, a liberal attitude to analgesia and/or sedation is required. We have found that pethidine or diamorphine infusions are particularly useful in this situation and that benzodiazepine sedation, for example with low doses of Hypnovel, is useful in the angiography suite.

Monitoring

Monitoring of patients is haematological/biochemical, clinical and radio-logical.

Baseline blood tests such as a full blood count, platelet count and clotting screen in the form of a prothrombin time and ratio plus a partial thromboplastin time (PTT) should be taken. These should be then monitored on a daily basis to follow the progress of the infusion. Any obvious defect in the initial clotting screen should be carefully considered before thrombolysis is undertaken and low haemoglobin or platelet count should be corrected before infusion begins. Should the haemoglobin drop without obvious cause on serial estimation, then retro-peritoneal haematoma should be suspected, particularly if a retroperitoneal Dacron graft is being lysed. This may be the only clinical sign of such a complication. A drop in haemoglobin of several grams/litre not infrequently happens without obvious cause. This is presumably due to blood loss into muscle and connective tissue in the treated limb. It can be surprisingly difficult to diagnose confidently in the absence of obvious skin bruising or the development of a compartment syndrome. This 'disappearing haemoglobin' phenomenon is well recognized by those with experience of thrombolysis, but as yet lacks a satisfactory explanation.

Fibrinogen levels and fibrin degradation products have been used in an attempt to predict haemorrhagic complications. Both these tests are non-specific, although a fibrinogen level of less than 1 g per litre has been correlated with haemorrhagic complications in some studies[4,5]. Excess thrombin generation during high-dose, systemic t-PA therapy has been reported[6]. This could theoretically cause a paradoxical hypercoagulable state and in the report cited was implicated in the possible aetiology of a myocardial infarction during systemic thrombolysis used to treat deep venous thrombosis.

The coagulation tests mentioned above are not generally available 24 hours a day and complications can occur even in the face of normal tests or while a test result is awaited. It would, therefore, appear imprudent to rely on them and in our view their current use is mainly for research. In the future, improved and more readily available markers of the coagulation and lytic pathways may appear. Monitoring of these markers would then become routine. Thromboelastography[7–9] has been used in liver transplantation and other circumstances where regular observation of clotting status is required. There is no data on its use in thrombolysis but it perhaps deserves consideration as a possible method of monitoring the coagulation disorder associated with thrombolytic infusions.

Reperfusion syndrome, if it occurs, will affect renal function and so a daily measurement of serum creatinine with urea and electrolytes is important. In high-risk patients, such as those with borderline limb viability or those who develop limb swelling or pain during treatment, the presence or absence of myoglobinuria should be sought and necessary treatment instigated to prevent renal failure. If severe, this may include amputation of the limb.

The mainstay of monitoring is radiology. Repeat angiographic examinations are necessary to follow the progress of low-dose thrombolysis and to reposition catheters as necessary. The timing of repeat angiography follows a standard pattern, but may need to be altered as determined by clinical monitoring. It is common to perform a check angiogram within 4 hours of the beginning of thrombolysis and at intervals from between 4 and 12 hours thereafter, depending on the clinical state of the limb.

Specific complications

Haemorrhage is the commonest complication of thrombolytic therapy, but is generally minor. Only a small proportion of patients experience major haemorrhage or stroke. In a review article in 1989[10], Berridge *et al.* drew attention to the fact that comparisons of haemorrhagic complications between different series were difficult because different criteria were used. They sensibly suggested that major haemorrhage should be defined as: haemorrhage requiring transfusion or causing hypotension or requiring specific treatment in the form of fresh frozen plasma, cryoprecipitate or antifibrinolytic drugs. We would suggest addition of a further category of major haemorrhage, namely, when even in the absence of the above factors a clinical decision was made to halt the thrombolytic infusion because of bleeding, as this has obvious prognostic significance for the limb (Table 7.3). Minor haemorrhage would be bleeding problems not fulfilling the above requirements. In Berridge's review, the results in 1401 patients treated with intra-arterial thrombolysis up to 1989 were collected[10]. The overall risk of stroke was 1%, major haemorrhage 5.1% and minor haemorrhage 14.8%. Therefore, approximately one in five patients will suffer a haemorrhage complication, but with only about a quarter of these being of great significance[4,10].

Haemorrhage

Puncture site bleeding and peri-catheter groin haematoma are related complications which depend on the size and number of vessel punctures and the agent used. Streptokinase with its longer half-life has been reported to cause more groin bleeding problems than other agents and this has been the experience in our hospital. Groin haematoma is caused by leakage of blood into the tissues around the arteriotomy site. It can be severe and require transfusion (Figure 7.3). Pain from groin haematoma can prevent adequate compression of the puncture site after repeat angiography and so predispose to further haemorrhage. Use of an introducer sheath (Figure 7.1), through which all catheter changes and manipulations are made, is very helpful in minimizing vessel trauma to decrease bleeding and haematoma formation. Adequate compression following catheter removal is important to ensure groin haematoma is kept to a minimum. Firm manual compression for a

Table 7.3 Definition of haemorrhagic complications during thrombolysis

Major haemorrhage
Haemorrhage —requiring blood transfusion
　　　　　　　—resulting in thrombolysis being halted prematurely
　　　　　　　—causing hypotention
　　　　　　　—requiring FFP, cryoprecipitate or antifibrinolytic drugs
　　　　　　　—fall in haemoglobin more than 5 g/dl
　　　　　　　—resulting in death

Minor haemorrhage
Haemorrhage which does not cause any of the above problems or require any specific therapy

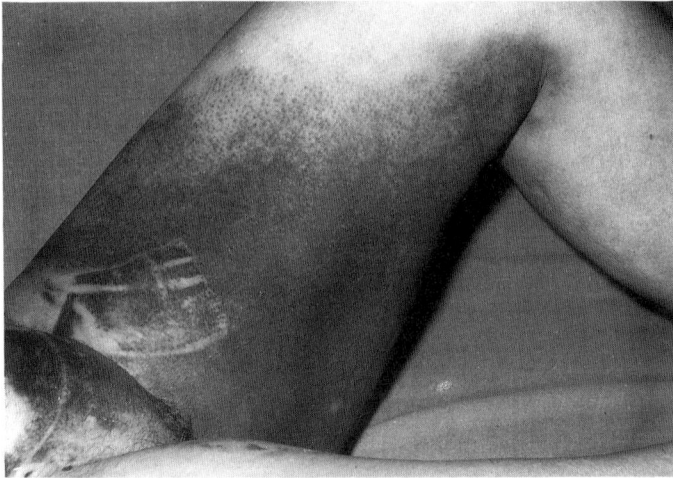

Figure 7.3 Pericatheter groin haematoma

period of 15–30 minutes is advised following catheter removal. This can then be followed by use of a compression dressing or sandbag for a variable period (<24 hours). Large groin haematoma can occasionally result in femoral nerve compression. Surgical evacuation may be helpful to prevent this problem.

The incidence of stroke with low-dose intra-arterial thrombolysis in our experience is about 2–5% (see later). This may be haemorrhagic or thrombotic and the two can be reliably differentiated by a contrast-enhanced CT scan (Figure 7.4). There is no way of predicting haemorrhagic stroke. Most authors consider 'recent stroke' a contraindication to thrombolysis but are less exact in the definition of 'recent'. A general consensus would be that a minimum period of 6 months is required before treatment with a thrombolytic drug should be considered. In our own experience a previous history of stroke did not predict stroke during thrombolysis. Close clinical monitoring as mentioned above, with prompt halting of the infusion, would appear to be the only way to limit intra-cranial bleeding. Fresh frozen plasma is readily available and should be given in the first instance if haemorrhagic stroke occurs. Cryoprecipitate is a more specific source of fibrinogen and is indicated for bleeding if fibrinogen levels are below 1 g/l. At least 12–18 units will be required. Non-haemorrhagic stroke can be due to either hypotension or to embolus. Hypotension may be caused by significant bleeding into lower limb muscles, a groin haematoma or inadvertent disconnection of arterial catheter lines. It may also be cardiac in origin. If hypotension is superimposed on cerebrovascular atheromatous disease, then the resultant loss of cerebral perfusion may lead to infarction. Prolonged hypotension should be avoidable by clinical monitoring.

Retroperitoneal haemorrhage is a potentially serious complication due to the large blood loss that can occur with minimal clinical signs. It has been described in relation to thrombolysis of retroperitoneal Dacron grafts but can occur whenever a groin puncture is used for thrombolysis. Many

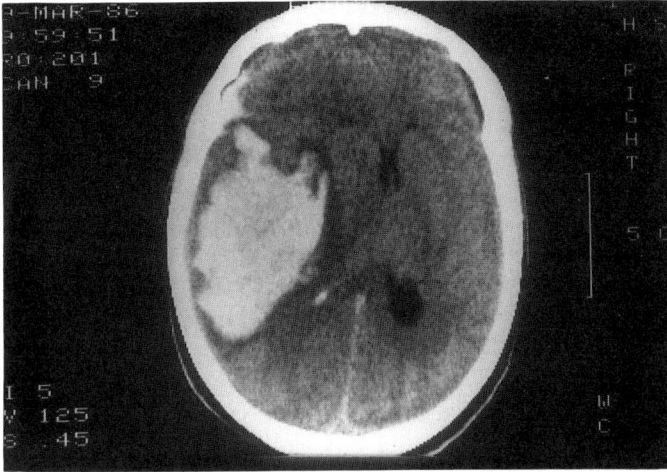

Figure 7.4 Contrast-enhanced CT brain scan revealing haemorrhagic stroke

retroperitoneal Dacron grafts have, however, been successfully and safely lysed and retroperitoneal haemorrhage is unusual in this situation. It seems likely that after 6 months the incorporation of retroperitoneal graft in fibrous tissue would preclude haemorrhage, although it is perhaps wise to undertake either ultrasound or CT scanning to ensure that there is no peri-graft seroma evident which might suggest failure of incorporation and into which haemorrhage could occur. Clinical observation for flank bleeding and daily haemoglobin levels to check for occult bleeding should minimize this complication. Paralytic ileus may be a feature of a large retroperitoneal haematoma. If there is clinical suspicion, the diagnosis of retroperitoneal haemorrhage will be made definitively by CT scanning.

Bleeding may rarely occur from other sites such as gastrointestinal haemorrhage, epistaxis or haematuria. Blood product support may be necessary with red cells, fresh frozen plasma or cryoprecipitate. If the bleeding is severe, then a decision must be made whether the infusion should be halted. This must be decided individually, with the dangers of a particular bleed weighed against the progress of the infusion and the threat to a limb. A major bleed will nearly always halt thrombolytic treatment, particularly if lysis is not well advanced, as the risk is to life rather than to limb.

Peri-catheter thrombus

A thin layer of thrombus may form along the length of the infusion catheter which is then sheared off into the arterial tree as the catheter is pulled back through the arterial wall during removal. If sufficiently large this clot may then lead to an immediate re-thrombosis. It has been traditional to use concomitant heparin therapy to prevent this, but it is not of proven benefit. We continue to use low-dose heparin (1000 units/hour) to prevent this complication. Infusion of a small dose of thrombolytic solution or heparin down the catheter side arm of an introducer sheath will bathe the upper parts of the infusion catheter and peri-catheter thrombus formation should be minimized. As the catheter is withdrawn the thrombus should collect within or around the tip of the introducer sheath where it will be lysed by the small dose of thrombolytic drug which we continue to infuse down the side arm of the sheath for up to 4 hours after withdrawal of the infusion catheter[2]. An alternative technique is slow withdrawal of the catheter while the infusion continues, so that sheared-off thrombus will be immediately lysed by the continuing infusion. This method has been favoured by the Nottingham group[11,12] (see Chapter 5).

Reperfusion syndrome

Reperfusion injury may be manifest in several forms such as sudden non-reversible deterioration in the limb or acute limb swelling, pain or respiratory distress, or renal failure with evidence of rhabdomyolysis. The injury is due to successful lysis of clot with reperfusion of a limb that has undergone some tissue necrosis. Toxic metabolites are washed back into the circulation with deleterious effects. Clinically this presents as increasing pain in the calf with loss of function and tenseness of the muscle compartment. Reperfusion oedema must be differentiated from small vessel embolization by repeat angiography where embolus will be obvious and compartment syndrome will be evident from slow flow within the affected tibial artery and extrinsic compression of the vessel branches. This problem should be preventable if correct evaluation of an ischaemic limb takes place initially. Recognition of reperfusion injury should be followed by prompt full-length fasciotomies to relieve muscle tension, excision of necrotic muscle and support of the respiratory or renal systems if required. Intravenous hydration will be necessary to maintain renal perfusion and in severe cases renal doses of inotropes will also be needed. Ventilation is not infrequently required to maintain tissue oxygenation. Despite these measures amputation and mortality in this group is high (see Chapter 2).

Distal embolization

Distal embolization occurs when the thrombolytic infusion softens up the thrombus, part of which then fragments and impacts further down the arterial tree (Figure 7.5). This occurs in about 12% of cases and the experience of UK centres in some 866 patients has recently been reviewed[13]. In the leg the embolus will commonly impact at the tibio-peroneal trunk and the effect is a sudden worsening of distal ischaemia during a successful thrombolytic infusion. The correct approach is to double the dose of thrombolytic agent and perform another contrast study quickly in order to re-position the catheter. It may be necessary to add an infusion through a hollow guide-wire positioned through the infusion catheter into the tibio-peroneal trunk and the general outcome is rapid lysis of this distal embolus. Catheter aspiration of clot may also be helpful. It is important to differentiate between a small amount of fresh thrombus which will quickly clear and a large volume of clot, e.g. from a popliteal aneurysm, which will completely occlude the run-off vessels and lead to acute, resistant limb deterioration. The incidence of this serious complication in a review of UK experience was 2%[13]. Urgent

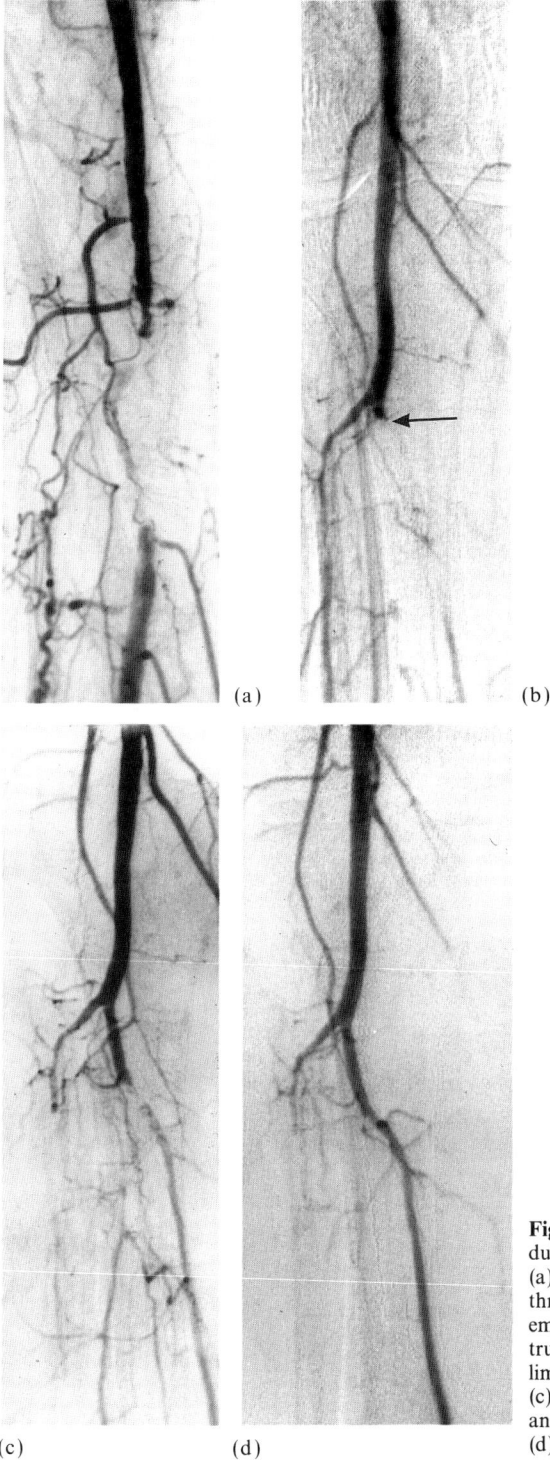

Figure 7.5 Distal embolization during thrombolysis.
(a) Superficial femoral artery thrombosis. (b) Distal embolization into tibio-peroneal trunk with sudden deterioration in limb perfusion (arrow)
(c) Catheter re-positioned distally and higher dose of t-PA infused.
(d) Distal embolus lysed

surgical exploration will then be needed to clear distal vessels and reconstruction may be required.

Allergic reactions

Allergic reactions are only described with streptokinase, an antigenic protein of bacterial origin. This is now much less common with modern preparations of the drug[14]. Allergy may happen as an anaphylactic reaction when the drug is first given and is probably related to previous streptococcal throat infections with subsequent antistreptococcal antibody formation. Skin rashes or serum sickness type allergic reactions are also seen[14,15]. Many patients will experience either allergy or diminished effect if streptokinase is used again within 6 months to 1 year. Co-administration of parenteral hydrocortisone is usual to cover repeated streptokinase therapy within these time limits. Allergic reactions are not seen with t-PA and are very rare with urokinase. The widespread use of systemic thrombolytic therapy for myocardial infarction and the fact that streptokinase is the most cost-effective agent means that many patients with vascular disease will have had exposure to streptokinase. It would therefore seem likely that the use of t-PA or urokinase in peripheral vascular occlusions will have much to offer in the avoidance of allergic complications in the future.

Arterial/graft perforation

Perforation of bypass grafts or native vessels with catheter guidewires is occasionally encountered (Figure 7.6). This will sometimes be of no great

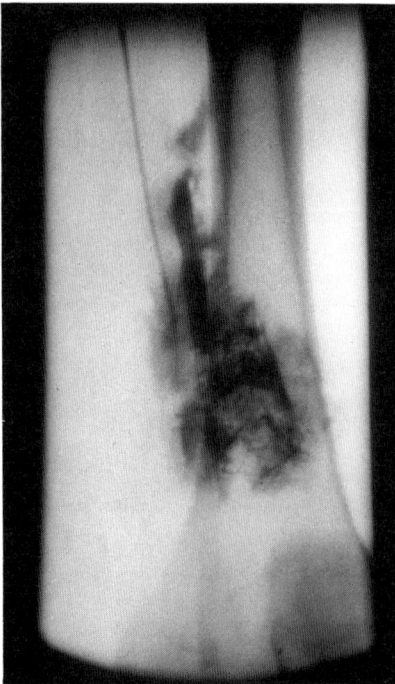

Figure 7.6 Graft perforation during thrombolysis causing contrast extravasation

significance and infusion can continue with successful results[16], but sometimes the perforation will be such that the thrombolytic infusion must be halted with potential lytic failure and limb loss. Occasionally, successful lysis of peripheral bypass grafts in the leg can cause bleeding from the lower end of the graft into the muscles of the calf. This again is usually insignificant and can be treated conservatively. Thrombolysis should be avoided in grafts which have been inserted within 7 days and it is best not used within 1 month of graft implantation. The failure of a bypass graft in the early post-operative period is usually due to a technical problem and should be treated by re-fashioning the graft, not by thrombolysis.

Catheter-related problems

Arterial spasm is a particular problem when catheters are situated within small, distal arteries, such as in the tibial vessels or within the arm. The problem appears to affect women more than men and is treated by intra-arterial injection of vasodilators, such as glyceryl trinitrate or nifedipine. It is probable that arterial spasm is also related to movement of the catheter and for this reason is likely to be minimized if the patient is immobile.

Audit

Meaningful alterations to practice can only be made if a careful audit of results is maintained and then compared to generally accepted results available in the medical literature. Units with an interest and experience in thrombolysis have recently agreed to the adoption of a common thrombolysis data record form to ensure uniform collection of national data (see Chapter 11). These data will then be centrally stored and should in the future provide very useful information concerning national practice. We have recently audited our own experience in the first 115 patients treated with thrombolysis at the Royal Free Hospital (Table 7.4).

In a detailed review of 115 patients, 61% were male and 39% female. The mean age of patients treated was 68.8 years with a range from 24 to 95 years. Interestingly, 25% of patients were aged 80 years or greater. The majority of patients (93/115) were treated with t-PA and the remainder with streptokinase.

Table 7.4 Audit of thrombolysis results ($n = 115$)

Result	%
Primary lytic success	70
Additional procedures	36
Major amputation	12
Stroke	4
Other haemorrhage	16
Mortality (30 days)	10

The indications for treatment were arterial thrombosis in 62%, graft failure in 26%, neglected embolus in 6%, venous thrombosis in 3% and popliteal aneurysm in 3%. Successful lysis was considered to have occurred if there was an anatomical and functional return either to normal, or to the pre-occlusive state following treatment. Re-establishment of run-off vessels with anatomical or adequate collateral supply was also considered to have been a success, as was meaningful graft salvage. The re-establishment of run-off vessels sufficient to allow a successful surgical bypass was also considered to be a good thrombolytic result. As defined above, there was successful lysis in 70% of cases with a primary lytic failure in 30%, which patients were then treated by other methods. Additional treatments were required in 35.6% of patients – 14.8% had an angioplasty, 5.2% benefited from in-flow surgery and 15.7% had distal reconstructions. In addition 8.7% of patients were placed on long-term anti-coagulation, fasciotomies were performed in 2.6% of patients and one patient had a sympathectomy.

There were 14 major amputations, five below knee and nine above knee: 11 of these 14 patients were alive and well at the time of this audit and three had died. There were four minor amputations, two of digits and two trans-metatarsal amputations, all of whom are alive and well. Complications included stroke in 4.3% of cases: one of these was haemorrhagic, two were due to embolus and two were due to hypotension. Three of the five patients who had a stroke during thrombolysis died. There was a 15.6% incidence of haemorrhage including puncture site bleeding, bleeding from peptic ulceration or local haematomas. Graft perforation occurred twice in the whole series. The mortality rate within 30 days was 10.4% (12 patients). Five patients died from cardiac arrest due to acute myocardial infarction, three died following stroke, two died from progressive limb ischaemia following lytic failure, one from lung cancer and one from a pulmonary embolus.

Previous audits of our earlier figures in this unit led us to abandon the use of streptokinase in favour of t-PA and also to use the catheter introducer sheath routinely in an attempt to prevent groin haematoma[3].

Conclusion

By selecting appropriate patients and treating them early in the evolution of their ischaemia, intra-arterial thrombolysis using a proven technique and a safe thrombolytic agent can be undertaken with minimal morbidity and mortality and an expectation of good overall results. Careful monitoring and clinical observation with a knowledge of the possible complications that can occur should also help minimize any iatrogenic morbidity. Avoidance of thrombolytic complications is an important determinant of patient outcome and also helps to maintain morale amongst the nursing, medical and radiology staff. This ensures an integrated and enthusiastic team approach which is essential for good overall results[17]. If successful lysis continues to be reported and the complications can be kept to a minimum, then it is to be expected that intra-arterial thrombolysis will continue to grow in popularity and become the dominant method for the treatment of acute vascular occlusion.

Acknowledgements

Dr A. Platts, Consultant Radiologist, Royal Free Hospital, for advice on the section concerning thrombolytic technique. Ms Isobel Smart, thrombolysis nurse specialist, Royal Free Hospital, for help with sections dealing with the nursing care and practical details of thrombolysis.

References

1. Hamilton G and Dawson K. Thrombolytic therapy for acute vascular emergencies. In: Greenhalgh RM, Hollier LH (eds) *Emergency Vascular Surgery*. Saunders, London, 1992; pp. 37–54
2. Dawson KJ, Reddy K, Platts AD and Hamilton G. Results of a recently instituted programme of thrombolytic therapy in acute lower limb ischaemia. *Br J Surg* 1991; **78**: 409–11
3. Dawson K, Dex E, Platts A and Hamilton G. Groin haemorrhage complicating intra-arterial thrombolytic therapy: choice of technique and agent. *Br J Surg* 1991; **78**: 363–4
4. Editorial. Non coronary thrombolysis. *Lancet* 1990; **335**: 691–3
5. Earnshaw JJ, Westby JC, Gregson RH, Makin GS and Hopkinson BR. Local thrombolytic therapy of acute peripheral arterial ischaemia with tissue plasminogen activator: a dose-ranging study. *Br J Surg* 1988; **75**: 1196–1200
6. Baglin TP, Luddington R, Jennings I and Richards EM. Thrombin generation and myocardial infarction during infusion of tissue-plasminogen activator. *Lancet* 1993; **341**: 504–5
7. Mallet SV, Cox D, Burroughs AK and Rolles K. The intra-operative use of trasylol (aprotinin) in liver transplantation. *Transplant Int* 1991; **4**: 227–30
8. Mallet SV and Cox D. Thromboelastography: the monitoring and treatment of coagulopathy during major surgery. *Br J Anaesth* 1992; **69**: 307–13
9. Mallet SV and Cox D. Thromboelastography: assessment of coagulation status and haemostatic therapy. *Care Crit Ill* 1993; **9**: 99–103
10. Berridge DC, Makin GS and Hopkinson BR. Local low dose intra-arterial thrombolytic therapy: the risk of stroke or major haemorrhage. *Br J Surg* 1989; **76**: 1230–33
11. Berridge DC, Gregson RH, Makin GS and Hopkinson BR. Tissue plasminogen activator in peripheral arterial thrombolysis. *Br J Surg* 1990; **77**: 179–82
12. Berridge DC, Gregson RH, Hopkinson BR and Makin GS. Intra-arterial thrombolysis using recombinant tissue plasminogen activator (r-TPA): the optimal agent, at the optimal dose? *Eur J Vasc Surg* 1989; **3**: 327–32
13. Galland RB, Earnshaw JJ, Baird RN, Lonsdale RJ, Hopkinson BR, Giddings AEB, Dawson KJ and Hamilton G. Acute limb deterioration during intra-arterial thrombolysis. *Br J Surg.* 1993, **80**: 1118–20
14. Earnshaw JJ. Thrombolytic therapy in the management of acute limb ischaemia. *Br J Surg* 1991; **78**: 261–9
15. Totty WM, Romano T, Benian GM, Gilula LA and Sherman LA. Serum sickness following streptokinase therapy. *Am J Roentgenol* 1982; **138**: 143–4
16. McCall J, Gleeson F, McGann G, Dawson K, Platts A and Hamilton G. Thrombolysis in high risk patients. *Clin Radiol* 1992; **45**: 298–301
17. Walker WJ and Giddings AEB. Thrombolysis – a challenge for radiologists and surgeons. *Clin Radiol* 1990; **41**: 299–300

Chapter 8

Thrombolytic agents

D. C. Berridge

Streptokinase

In 1933, Tillett and Garner working in the Rockefeller Institute reported that filtrates of beta haemolytic streptococci caused rapid liquefaction of human plasma coagulum[1]. Further investigation led to an understanding of the mechanism of streptococcal fibrinolysis. Christensen[2] demonstrated that the strepto-coccus produces an activator or kinase, a single protein of approximately 47 000 molecular weight.

Streptokinase forms an equimolar complex with plasminogen after overcoming the effect of antibodies present in the circulation, the result of previous streptococcal infection[3,4]. The bound plasminogen then undergoes a transition, and exposes an active site in the modified plasminogen moiety, the complex becoming a potent plasminogen activator. The biological half-life of streptokinase is approximately 30 minutes.

The addition of small amounts of streptokinase to a given quantity of plasminogen produces a high level of plasmin (dependent on the time allowed for activation). In contrast, high concentrations of streptokinase produce little plasmin and a high level of activator. Maximum activity is obtained when streptokinase and plasminogen exist in approximately equal proportions.

Despite the comparatively low dose used in peripheral arterial thrombolysis, a progressive systemic response is still seen with streptokinase at a dose of 5000 units per hour after 4 hours. This effect is also seen with t-PA but is significantly reduced and occurs later than with streptokinase[5].

Repeat treatment with streptokinase is unpredictable due to a sustained rise in anti-streptococcal antibodies which occurs in most patients. Extremely large doses would be needed to counteract this effect with subsequent unpredictable results and a possible increase in haemorrhagic complications[6]. The anti-streptococcal titre was thought to return to normal after approximately 4–6 months[7]. However, Elliott *et al.* have followed up 145 patients who received 1.5 million units of streptokinase for coronary thrombolysis between 11 and 48 months previously. They found that antibody titres sufficient to neutralize a conventional dose of 1.5 million units streptokinase were present in 50% after 2 years, 52% after 3 years and 49% after 4 years[8]. Hence streptokinase and related compounds such as anistreplase could be ineffective for up to 4 years following an initial administration. In the absence of anti-streptococcal antibodies, the plasma half-life of streptokinase is approximately 18 minutes. However, when antibodies are present this is considerably extended to 83 minutes *in vitro*[9].

Pyrexia occurs in about one-third of patients who receive streptokinase, with 5% experiencing a temperature in excess of 104°F[10]. This is currently much less of a problem than in earlier years due to the increased purity of the streptokinase. Severe anaphylactic reactions, although rare, can be fatal[11]. Allergic reactions occur in up to 20% of people treated with streptokinase, but are usually mild. Apart from stopping the infusion itself, the use of bronchodilators, antihistamines and large doses of steroids are used as required[12]. Administration of corticosteroids prior to streptokinase therapy may prevent febrile reactions but usually treatment with paracetamol is sufficient.

In addition to its thrombolytic effect, streptokinase reduces blood and plasma viscosities, and red cell aggregation. These effects are primarily due to a significant reduction in plasma fibrinogen concentration, and may account for the symptomatic improvement in patients with deep venous thrombosis or a myocardial infarction, prior to any thrombolytic effect being apparent[13].

Even with small doses of streptokinase, a significant anticoagulant effect is produced. Large doses of streptokinase will deplete plasminogen, reducing the fibrinolytic potential of the blood. If rethrombosis occurs at this stage, the thrombus formed may contain only small amounts of plasminogen and be less susceptible to further attempts at lysis. Streptokinase can also exert a significant pro-aggregatory platelet effect both *in vitro* and *ex vivo*[14–16]. Increased platelet degradation products have been reported post coronary thrombolysis for acute myocardial infarction[17].

At the conclusion of fibrinolytic treatment with streptokinase, a rebound thrombotic effect may increase the risk of rethrombosis, hence streptokinase therapy should always be followed initially by anticoagulation with heparin.

Urokinase

MacFarlane and Pilling first drew attention to the presence of fibrinolytic activity in human urine[18–20].

Urokinase is a trypsin-like protease composed of two polypeptide chains (molecular weights, 20 000 and 34 000 respectively), connected by a single disulfide bond. It can be extracted from human urine, but can also be produced by kidney cells in culture[21]. It converts plasminogen directly into plasmin but, unlike streptokinase, it does not require an intermediate proactivator. The biological half-life of urokinase is approximately 10–15 minutes[22]. It is non-antigenic and less toxic than streptokinase but more expensive to produce. Furthermore, there are no anti-urokinase antibodies in human plasma, hence a fixed dose regimen can be used. Cragg studied two different urokinase dose regimens in a prospective randomized trial[23]. Patients received either 250 000 units (u) per hour for 4 hours followed by 125 000 u per hour, or a low-dose infusion of 50 000 u per hour. The rate of major complications was similar, though minor bleeding complications were more frequent in the high-dose group. The low-dose regimen was equally effective in achieving successful peripheral arterial thrombolysis.

According to van Breda and Katzen[24] and McNamara and Fischer[25], the use of urokinase in local low-dose peripheral arterial thrombolysis is associated with improved lysis and reduced haemorrhagic complications associated with a reduced systemic effect when compared with streptokinase. This viewpoint is widely held in North America.

New fibrin-specific thrombolytic agents

Pro-urokinase (scu-PA)

Although urokinase was isolated from urine in 1954, pro-urokinase, its inactive precursor, remained unknown until 1977. Nolan et al. observed a plasminogen activator in human embryonic kidney cell cultures which reacted with anti-urokinase antibodies but could be separated from urokinase by chromatography on benzamidine-sepharose – 'a pro-activator of urokinase' or pro-urokinase[26]. It is presently termed single chain urokinase plasminogen activator (scu-PA) and may be manufactured by recombinant DNA technology.

Scu-PA can be distinguished from urokinase by its properties – a higher fibrin specificity and lower activity, and by its single chain structure[27]. Collen et al. demonstrated in vivo that scu-PA was superior to urokinase in fibrin specificity and thrombolytic efficacy[28]. Gurewich evaluated the relative potency of urokinase and scu-PA in rabbits and dogs with experimentally induced pulmonary emboli[29,30]. He observed 6%, 17% and 53% lysis with saline, urokinase and scu-PA respectively. In blood, scu-PA is present in approximately the same concentrations as tissue-type plasminogen activator (t-PA). Although t-PA is about ten times as potent, scu-PA retains its activity for at least 24 hours in contrast to urokinase which is inactivated within a few hours[31]. The stability of scu-PA is dependent upon the concentration of plasma inhibitors, as shown in buffered saline solution where highly purified scu-PA can activate plasminogen (albeit slowly), and then in turn be activated by the plasmin produced[30]. Plasminogen activated by scu-PA appears to change shape when bound to fibrin. This is different from plasminogen activated by t-PA which appears to be bound to an internal lysine binding site on fibrin. t-PA and scu-PA appear to activate different fibrin-bound plasminogens, and hence act synergistically when administered together[31].

During thrombolysis, scu-PA is progressively converted to urokinase. As urokinase is more reactive this results in an acceleration of plasminogen activation[31]. Another important property of pro-urokinase is its ability to lyse platelet rich clots. Platelets promote the fibrinolytic effect of scu-PA but not t-PA in vitro.

As yet, scu-PA has not been evaluated in peripheral arterial ischaemia. Early results for coronary thrombolysis are encouraging. The special properties of scu-PA promote optimism and results of its use in peripheral thrombolysis are anticipated with interest.

Anistreplase (acylated-plasminogen-streptokinase-activator complex)

In an attempt to reduce the frequency of haemorrhagic complications and in particular stroke, whilst maintaining or improving success rates, the search has continued for synthetic fibrin-specific agents.

Various acylated derivatives of streptokinase have been produced[32]. The most studied is anistreplase, an acylated complex of streptokinase and plasminogen (Eminase, SmithKline Beecham Pharmaceuticals). Anistreplase is produced by locating an acyl group on the catalytic side of the enzyme. The compound itself has no thrombolytic properties. Following fibrin binding, deacylation occurs and results in activation of the agent. The result is an enhanced concentration of activator complex bound to fibrin. The major advantage of anistreplase is that it is easily administered intravenously in a bolus injection regimen every 8 hours[33]. Its biological half-life following intravenous bolus ad-ministration is approximately 100 minutes[22]. Unlike *in vitro* data, most clinical studies have not confirmed specificity for fibrin but reveal that anistreplase is associated with a variable systemic fibrino-genolytic effect, although this is generally less than either streptokinase or urokinase[34,35]. Its use in peripheral arterial thrombolysis was associated with low limb salvage and high complication rates[36]. Anistreplase has never been tested by the intra-arterial route in acute leg ischaemia where it should have no advantage over streptokinase. It may, however, find a role as a useful alternative in myocardial infarction.

Tissue plasminogen activator (t-PA)

t-PA was first discovered using a cadaver isolated limb perfusion model, and was subsequently purified by Binder[37]. Rijken in 1979 was able to extract 1 mg of t-PA from 5 kg of human uterine tissue[38]. Further development, and in particular the ability to perform clinical trials, only became feasible with the advent of a far richer source of t-PA – a human melanoma cell culture line[39] – and subsequently with the development of recombinant t-PA using DNA technology[40,41]. Initial production of t-PA was a small-scale process and resulted in between 1% and 5% single chain and the remainder two-chain t-PA. After scaling up to a commercially viable process, production became predominantly single chain t-PA (70–80%). Although the kinetics of the two types of t-PA differ, there are no significant differences in thrombolytic properties, or fibrin specificity.

In the absence of fibrin, t-PA is only a weak plasminogen activator. In the presence of fibrin, a 500–1000 fold increase in activation occurs. t-PA has a half-life of 5–7 minutes in the presence of fibrin. This is primarily due to an affinity of fibrin-bound t-PA for plasminogen which does not influence the catalytic efficiency of plasminogen binding to fibrin. Furthermore, t-PA enhances plasminogen binding to fibrin[42]. The summation of these properties is a relatively 'fibrin specific' effect, achieving local lysis with a reduced systemic effect. In local low-dose administration of t-PA, plasminogen activation is also facilitated because fibrin-bound plasmin is relatively resistant to inhibition by alpha-2-antiplasmin[43]. *In vitro* clot-lysis studies have shown that t-PA is approximately 5–10 times more effective than urokinase[44,45], without inducing fibrinogenolysis and with only a modest reduction in plasminogen and alpha-2-antiplasmin.

The first clinical case report used melanoma derived t-PA in a renal allograft recipient who developed a massive renal and ilio-femoral vein thrombosis. An intravenous dose of 7.5 mg over 24 hours achieved successful lysis[46].

In a recent randomized study in peripheral arterial thrombolysis there

were significant advantages of intra-arterial t-PA over intra-arterial streptokinase therapy with regard to radiologically demonstrated lysis, amputation
rate and the increase in ankle/brachial pressure index (Tables 8.1–8.3)[47].
Similarly there were significantly fewer haemorrhagic complications with
intra-arterial t-PA than with intra-arterial streptokinase. These results
therefore appear to confirm increased efficacy and safety of locally administered
t-PA over streptokinase in this study.

A further advantage of t-PA is its non-antigenicity and hence repeated
doses are feasible without risk of allergic complications or indeed the
unpredictability of second streptokinase administrations with the profound

Table 8.1 Randomized trial of thrombolysis: results

	Agent		
	IA Streptokinase	IA t-PA	IV t-PA
Patients	20	20	20
Radiological			
Success	16 (80%)	20 (100%)*	9 (45%)
Failure	4	0	11
Angioplasty	4	8	1
Clinical improvement	16 (80%)	20 (100%)	11 (55%)
Increase in ABI			
Median	0.24	0.57**	0.18
Range	(0–0.57)	(0.33–0.82)	(0–0.41)

* $0.01 < P < 0.04$ ⎫ compared to other two groups.
** $P < 0.001$ ⎭

Reproduced from Berridge et al. Br J Surg 1991; **78**: 988–95, by permission of the publishers, Butterworth-Heinemann Ltd.

Table 8.2 Randomised trial of thrombolysis: outcome

	Agent		
	IA Streptokinase	IA t-PA	IV t-PA
30-day limb salvage:			
Asymptomatic	12 (60%)	16 (80%)	9 (45%)
Critical ischaemia	0	0	5
Amputation	7	1	0
Death	1 pneumonia	1 pneunomia	2 pneumonia
		2 myocardial infarction	1 myocardial infarction
Reconstructed or	0	0	2
IA lysis	0	0	1
3-month limb salvage			
Asymptomatic	12 (60%)	15 (75%)	10 (50%)
Critical ischaemia	0	0	1
Amputation	6	1	1
Death	2	4	5

Reproduced from Berridge et al. Br J Surg 1991; **78**: 988–95, by permission of the publishers, Butterworth-Heinemann Ltd.

Table 8.3 Randomized trial of thrombolysis: complications

	Agent		
	IA Streptokinase	*IA t-PA*	*IV t-PA*
CVA	0	0	1
Haemorrhage			
Major	3	0	3
Minor	3	0	9
Perforation	0	1	0
Rethrombosis	4	2	0
Embolization	0	1	0

Reproduced from Berridge *et al. Br J Surg* 1991; **78**: 988–95, by permission of the publishers, Butterworth-Heinemann Ltd.

antibody response that prevails. In blood samples from over 700 patients treated with t-PA worldwide, only three gave positive results for detection of antibodies to t-PA by a radioimmunoprecipitation assay. None of these cases had neutralizing antibodies, and in each case, subsequent samples evaluated between 3 weeks and 10 months after treatment proved negative[48].

The search for an ideal thrombolytic agent

It is illogical to assume that the most fibrin-specific 'ideal' agent will be free from all risk of stroke and haemorrhage. Patients will continue to have silent strokes and asymptomatic or unrecognized peptic ulceration in association with a haemostatic platelet-thrombus plug. The ideal agent can only recognize these as 'legitimate' targets. It will therefore lyse this plug as readily as it will the peripheral arterial thrombus it was intended to treat. The relative maturity of the thrombus will determine when, and if, the complication will occur. For example, when thrombolytic agents are used for thrombosis of Dacron grafts, massive haemorrhage occasionally ensues. Dacron grafts, particularly if knitted, may never be covered fully with neointima, and their integrity relies on thrombus incorporated in the interstices of the graft. Providing the dose of the lytic agent is either high enough or is administered for long enough, leakage should not be unexpected[49,50]. Fibrin specificity may not be the most important property of a successful thrombolytic drug. Meanwhile the search continues and presently monoclonal antifibrin antibody bound agents look an attractive proposition for the future.

Relative fibrinolytic effects of thrombolytic agents

All thrombolytic agents cause a degree of systemic fibrinolysis which is dose specific. The individual effect is dependent on the fibrin-binding properties of the agent and the level of inhibitors or antibodies. Unfortunately the effects are often rather unpredictable.

Intravenous administration of high doses of either streptokinase or urokinase results in a plasminogen level of less than 1% of normal within 4 hours which remains at 0.5% for the duration of the infusion[51,52]. This recovers to approximately 50% of the initial level within 24 hours of completing the infusion. As lysis is dependent not only on the plasminogen contained within the thrombus but also within the plasma, this can limit the efficacy of the lytic agent.

Plasma fibrinogen is profoundly depleted to approximately 1.5 g/l or lower during treatment. Fibrin and fibrinogen degradation products (FDP) rise within 4 hours due to a combination of fibrin degradation within the thrombus and degradation of circulating plasma fibrinogen. The haemorrhagic risk is exacerbated by the combination of high FDPs which themselves are anticoagulant, and low fibrinogen.

t-PA has comparatively little systemic effect when given as a rapid bolus infusion for coronary thrombolysis[53]. If prompt lysis of a large thrombus occurs, the FDPs will inevitably rise, and excessive elevation of FDPs has been reported after coronary thrombolysis using t-PA.

The advent of fibrin-specific agents was hailed as a major breakthrough enabling intravenous administration; however, clinical experience was unfortunately less satisfactory. Anistreplase had a high risk of major haemorrhage and even death, associated with a poor lysis rate[36]. Recombinant t-PA gave further hope, with little circulating plasminogen; naturally existing inhibitors such as alpha-2-antiplasmin effectively neutralize its action *in vivo*. Hence the action of t-PA is concentrated locally onto fibrin-bound plasminogen[54]. On a molar basis, t-PA is a more effective lytic agent than either streptokinase or urokinase. Both streptokinase and urokinase produced higher fibrinogenolysis (60% and 50% respectively) than the 20% associated with t-PA[45]. Although a systemic effect is still seen with t-PA, this is significantly less than with streptokinase in the same situation[5].

Synergistic effects

Gurewich and Pannell have demonstrated a marked synergistic effect using a combination of t-PA and scu-PA[30]. Similar findings have also been reported by Collen et al.[55]. In a rabbit jugular vein model, significantly enhanced thrombolysis was seen during the simultaneous infusion of t-PA with scu-PA and t-PA with urokinase, but not scu-PA with urokinase, than could be anticipated on the basis of the added effects of each agent alone. Preliminary results in patients with myocardial infarction confirmed that combined administration of t-PA and scu-PA, in doses lower than normally used, resulted in equivalent lysis but no associated systemic fibrinogenolysis[56].

Comparison of clinical effects of thrombolytic agents

Comparison between clinical trials of thrombolytic agents is very difficult as there is widespread variation in site, length and age of arterial occlusion. The different proportions of graft thrombosis compared with native vessel occlusions render direct comparison almost impossible. The age of occlusion can vary widely in different reports, ranging from a mean of 18 days (range 1–60)[47], whilst in other studies it was 7 days[57] and 14 days[36]. Similarly patients over 70 years of age may have a poorer response[58]. The mean age in our randomized trial was 75.3 years compared to 59.6 years in a study from the Cleveland Clinic, USA[57]. This may explain the shorter duration of therapy required and the ability to cope with the much higher dose of t-PA used in the latter study (effectively 3.5–7 mg per hour for a 70 kg patient).

Systemic administration of t-PA has been shown to be of value in coronary thrombolysis[59–61]. In peripheral arterial thrombolysis, the length of the occlusion and volume of thrombus, the diameter of the vessel and the duration of history are all considerably greater. Hence short-duration, high-dose thrombolysis is unlikely to achieve the same success if applied to peripheral arterial thromboses. If systemic thrombolysis is considered for peripheral arterial thromboses, a fibrin-specific agent is needed which can be given over several hours without incurring a profound systemic lytic effect. Results obtained from the coronary thrombolysis studies must be interpreted with caution before extrapolating them to the field of peripheral arterial thrombolysis.

Urokinase vs streptokinase

In a retrospective analysis of 47 patients receiving either urokinase or streptokinase, van Breda et al. compared the efficacy of lysis, the degree of systemic thrombolytic effect, and the rate of complications[24]. They concluded that the overall efficacy was superior in the urokinase group (80%). Streptococcal antibody titres were measured in all patients. Patients with high titres who subsequently received streptokinase, responded poorly (20% lysis). These same patients obtained successful lysis with urokinase. Streptokinase was also shown to produce a more marked effect on fibrinogen levels and thrombin time. In the streptokinase group the incidence of bleeding complications was 33% compared to 8% in the urokinase group.

Similarly, Gardiner reported 72 thrombosed peripheral arterial grafts in 62 patients treated by either intra-arterial urokinase or intra-arterial streptokinase. Urokinase was associated with an 84% (43 cases) success rate compared to 45% (29 cases) in the streptokinase group[62]. Ultimately, however, a successful outcome depends on finding an underlying aetiological factor which can be corrected. In 25 patients with an underlying stenosis which could be angioplastied, the 1 year patency was 86%. This was in contrast to 25 grafts where no underlying stenosis was seen in which the 1 year patency was 37%.

Using high-dose urokinase, McNamara and Fischer demonstrated an 83% lysis rate in association with a 4% incidence of major haemorrhage[25]. These results are not dissimilar to those obtained with low-dose streptokinase[63], despite being in a younger population (mean age 59 years) and with 72 of 83 lesions (87%) of less than 10 days' duration. Furthermore 10 patients had thrombosed arterio-venous dialysis shunts, but insufficient data were provided to allow separation of this good prognosis group from those with lower limb thromboembolism[25].

t-PA vs streptokinase

In a recent randomized study including 40 patients, intra-arterial t-PA offered a 20% (confidence limits: 8% to 48%) increase in limb salvage at 30 days over conventional therapy with streptokinase although this did not achieve statistical significance (Tables 8.1–8.3)[47]. Radiological lysis, increase in ankle-brachial indices and haemorrhagic complications were all significantly improved with t-PA.

Comparison with other regimens in different centres is often difficult due to large population differences, and also the inclusion of multiple indications including haemodialysis fistulae which have a totally different prognosis from that of lower limb thromboembolism[57,64]. Using streptokinase, Graor et al. achieved an initial patency rate of 55% in thrombosed lower limb arteries[57]. This same group at the Cleveland Clinic, USA later published improved results using t-PA, with complete thrombolysis occurring in 20 (95%) patients[65]. Unfortunately no data are given with regard to the mean age of the patients, or the duration of ischaemia. Nevertheless, results from the latest Cleveland study show an equally favourable response using t-PA at a lower dose (0.05–0.1 mg/kg/h)[65]. Encouraging results have also been reported by Verstraete using comparatively high doses of t-PA, with an initial patency of up to 94%, but with a higher incidence of haemorrhagic complications (37%)[66]. Hence lower doses such as used in the Nottingham study (0.5 mg/h) appear to offer a similar thrombolytic success rate, with fewer complications[47].

In a large audit of peripheral arterial thrombolysis, the Nottingham group concluded that t-PA was superior to streptokinase in rate of lysis (58% vs 41%) and also significantly reduced the required duration of lysis (22 hours vs 40 hours)[67]. However, it should be noted that there was no overall difference in the frequency of haemorrhagic complications, although many were encountered during an early dose ranging study of t-PA[58]. A recent non-randomized comparative series failed to show any significant advantage using t-PA[68]. Although initial pooled results did not show any reduction in haemorrhagic complications with t-PA, it is noted that clinicians now appear to be using lower doses.[69]

Whereas streptokinase is associated with a pro-aggregatory platelet effect. t-PA has been shown to inhibit platelet aggregation, and may even result in disaggregation.[70] To achieve a clinically significant effect, it is suggested that co-administration of t-PA and a platelet antagonist may enhance thrombolysis[71]. It is possible that haemorrhagic complications occurring with t-PA may be due to its plasmin-mediated effects on platelets which result in a significant increase in template bleeding time within 90 minutes of infusion.

Intravenous administration of t-PA for peripheral arterial thrombolysis was disappointing. Poor lysis was attended by a high incidence of haemorrhagic complications including one stroke[47]. The relative 'fibrin-specificity' of t-PA was compromised by systemic administration probably due to the higher doses required, which resulted in an intermediate effect on systemic activation. Accordingly the haemorrhagic complications were more frequent than with low-dose intra-arterial t-PA. Complications were due to a combination of lysis of the 'sealing' thrombus at venepuncture sites and also to the increased systemic lytic state as reflected in the shorter euglobulin lysis time.

t-PA vs urokinase

Meyerovitz et al. performed a randomized study of t-PA and urokinase[72]. The t-PA was administered as a 10 mg bolus, then at 5 mg/h for up to 24

Table 8.4 Randomized comparison of t-PA and urokinase in peripheral thrombolysis

Time (h)	No. of patients studied		*Cumulative no. of patients with 95% lysis and restitution of antegrade flow*		
	t-PA*	*Urokinase†*	*t-PA* (n = 16)	*Urokinase* (n = 16)	*P Value‡*
4	16	16	4 (25)	0 (0)	0.10
8	10	11	7 (44)	1 (6)	0.04
16	1	4	7 (44)	3 (19)	0.25
24	5	10	8 (50)	6 (38)	0.72

Reproduced with permission from Meyerovitz *et al. Radiology* 1990; **175**: 75–8.

Note, Percentages are in parentheses.
* One patient was not studied beyond 4 hours because of termination of t-PA infusion after apparent extravasation on the 4 hour arteriogram (later found to be a pseudoaneurysm); three patients were not studied at 24 hours because t-PA infusion was terminated after bleeding occurred.
† One patient was not studied beyond 4 hours because of termination of urokinase infusion after bleeding occurred; two patients were not studied at 24 hours because of premature termination of urokinase infusion by the angiographer (one was a protocol violation at 16.5 hours; the other patient was believed to have marked clot lysis at 8 hours, but this was refuted by the blind panel of investigators).
‡ Fisher exact test.

hours (total dose 135 mg, cost £1645). Urokinase was administered as a 60 000 iu bolus, then 240 000 iu/h for 2 hours, 129 000 iu/h for 2 hours and finally 60 000 iu/h for up to 20 hours (total dose 1 988 000 iu, cost £1350). t-PA produced a higher rate of lysis in a shorter duration (Table 8.4). However, possibly due to small numbers, statistical significance was not reached. Nevertheless, there did appear to be a trend in favour of t-PA.

Cost-effectiveness of thrombolysis

Information required to ascertain the cost-effectiveness of procedures is distinctly lacking in all aspects of vascular surgery, including the field of peripheral arterial thrombolysis. A recent evaluation of surgery for critical leg ischaemia at St Mary's Hospital, London showed that distal vascular reconstruction was cost effective in terms of limb salvage, but more importantly in the improved mobility of patients, within the home and outside[73]. The high cost of caring for amputees is justification for the time and money spent on vascular surgery for limb salvage. The same argument may be used for thrombolysis in acute leg ischaemia.

For specific indications, e.g. popliteal aneurysms, graft thromboses, distal emboli, the very ill and patients with poor run off, peripheral arterial thrombolysis is certainly a viable option. However, to be cost effective, initial lysis must be as durable and have similar complications to surgery.

Hess has reported an early re-thrombosis rate of 25% after thrombolysis; however, of those functioning at 2 weeks, 70% remain patent at 1 year and 65% patent at 5 years[74]. Similarly, Lammer reported a 10% early re-thrombosis rate with 81% patency at 2 years[75]. These figures compare favourably with those obtained for femoro-distal surgery for critical ischaemia.

Tissue plasminogen
  activator   Streptokinase
_____   _____

                                                              Antigenic – Allergenic
                                                                        – Anaphylaxis
                                                              Proaggregatory – effects
                                                              Single use only
           Expensive   Anti-Sk antibodies

           Non-antigenic   Cheap
           Rapid lysis
           Anti-platelet effects
           More complete lysis
           Less systemic effect
           Repeatable

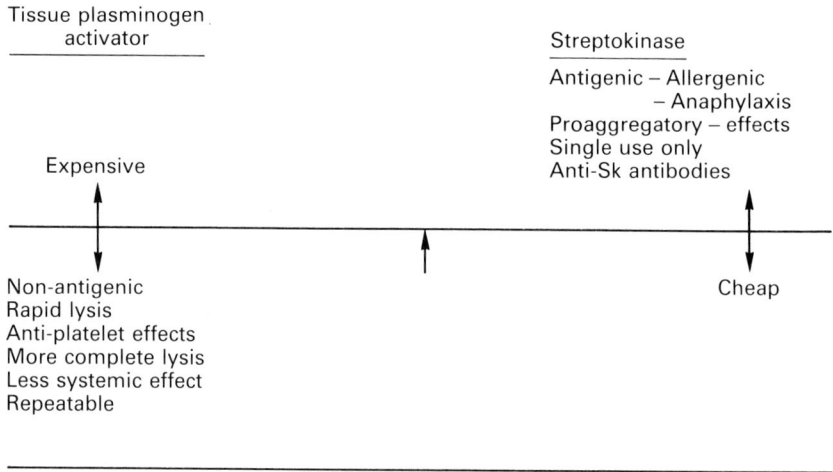

Figure 8.1 The optimal thrombolytic agent?

Cost was considered to be a major factor in limiting use of thrombolysis in 3% of respondents in a recent questionnaire[76], though other factors such as allergic reactions and haemorrhagic risk must all be taken into the equation when balancing the relative benefits of thrombolysis (Figure 8.1).

Measurement of cost-effectiveness

Peripheral arterial thrombolysis is a labour-intensive treatment, especially when used in a low-dose regimen. Constant surveillance and adjustments in catheter position/angioplasty, reviewing the need for surgical intervention and general medical care, ensure a major commitment for the surgeon and interventional radiologist. Other 'hidden' costs are the need for closer nursing support and the services of a radiographer. In a busy hospital it could be difficult to find extra resources to run a thrombolysis service. However, this vigilance is probably no more than would be expected for the post-operative care of a patient following a femoro-distal graft.

Published information about the cost-effectiveness of intra-arterial thrombolysis is limited. Dacey et al. reported 24 infusions in 23 patients over a 4-year period (i.e. six patients per year)[77]. A combination of drugs was used in a non-randomized manner. Although five (21%) patients were classified as complete success, in a further seven (29%) surgery was avoided, limited or postponed, i.e. lysis was beneficial. Five (25%) patients deteriorated and required urgent surgery.

Although costs were calculated in this study, they are subject to debate. For example, costs of $2399 were associated with thrombolytic medications. The drugs used were either streptokinase ($114) or urokinase ($3451). A mean cost for thrombolytic therapy was then calculated – clearly an overestimate for the patients who received streptokinase. In this study, the cost per case for completely or partially successful thrombolysis was $16 500. If streptokinase or even t-PA had been used this cost would have been lower.

Finally no allowance was made for the possible improvement in run-off or freeing/fragmenting of thrombus that may have occurred in patients due to earlier thrombolysis who later required surgery, which might have improved subsequent outcome. As Dacey points out 'better patient selection might improve the success rate', and therefore improve the cost-effectiveness of the technique.

Graor et al. compared thrombolysis of occluded peripheral arterial grafts to surgical thrombectomy[78]. In a case-controlled comparison of 22 patients undergoing thrombolysis and 38 patients undergoing surgical thrombectomy, 91% of t-PA treated patients required a secondary procedure to maintain arterial patency. Similarly 89% of surgically treated patients required graft revision. The surgical group had a three-fold increased risk of amputation. Graor stated that speedier lysis was possible with t-PA (4–5 hours) compared to urokinase (12–24 hours). The advantage of thrombolysis was that it could lyse thrombus in tibial and more distal arteries that could not be removed surgically, thereby allowing a lower resistance vascular bed. Superior results were obtained with lysis plus surgery than with surgery alone.

Janosik et al. compared streptokinase, urokinase and surgical thrombectomy retrospectively in a non-randomized study of graft occlusions (Table 8.5)[79]. In 19 administrations using streptokinase, seven were successful though one re-occluded within 60 days to give a cumulative success rate of 32%. Urokinase was used on 23 occasions in 18 patients. Fifteen had success with one re-occlusion within 60 days to give a cumulative success rate of 64%. Cumulative patency in the surgical thrombectomy group was 76%. The higher efficacy of urokinase has to be tempered with its higher cost. It should be noted that no allowance is made for the difference in costs after hospital discharge.

Is t-PA 'worth' an extra £180–200 per patient? Walker and Giddings report very good results using streptokinase alone[63]. Hence the added benefit of t-PA might be small. However, both in the randomized study and in the larger prospective audit from Nottingham, the increased efficacy and reduced complications would appear to justify the added expense of t-PA[47,67]. Earnshaw et al. were unable to demonstrate improved results after they changed from routine use of streptokinase to t-PA[68] in a sequential study.

Selection is obviously the key to cost-effective treatment. Poor selection leads to poor results, high complication rates and high costs. The overall cost of an admission for acute leg ischaemia is great and differences in cost of the thrombolytic agent are largely irrelevant. Consider other comparative

Table 8.5 Comparison of methods of treatment for graft thrombosis

Treatment group	Length of stay (days)	Thrombolytic agent	Total hospital charges
Thrombectomy	21.1	—	$25 336
Streptokinase	21.3	$690*	$25 978
Urokinase	11.5†	$6429*	$22 203

Reproduced with permission from Janosik et al. Invest Radiol 1991; **26**: 921–5.

* $P < 0.001$.
† $P < 0.05$.

Table 8.6 Approximate costs of materials for thrombolysis and surgery

Material/device	Cost
Femoro-popliteal graft (PTFE 60 cm 6 mm)	£730
Fogarty embolectomy catheter	
2F	£62
5F	£27
Angioplasty catheter 5F	£105
Angioplasty catheter ultra-thin 5F	£150
Thrombolytic agents	
Streptokinase (Kabikinase, Kabi/Knowlhill)	
100 000 u	£8.31
20 h course (5000 u/h)	£8.31
Recombinant tissue plasminogen activator (Boerhinger Ingelheim, Bracknell)	
20 mg	
20 h course (1 mg/h)	£176.00
Urokinase (Serono, Welwyn Garden City)	£60.00
100 000 u	
20 h course*	£1054

Note: Costs may vary depending on locally negotiated prices.
* Urokinase 60 000 u bolus, 240 000 u/h for 2 h, 129 000 u/h for 2 h, finally 60 000 u for 16 h.

costs such as prosthetic material for other vascular reconstructive procedures (Table 8.6). Formal cost-benefit analysis of any vascular procedure needs to include not just hospital costs, but also overall costs up to and including full rehabilitation. Costs attributed to hospital stay, rehabilitation for both patients with limb salvage and amputees, community care costs and functional tests for both groups need to be included.

The cost of amputation has been calculated at approximately £30 000 per year compared to approximately £1000 per year after successful vascular reconstruction[80]. However, Fyfe suggests that these figures may in reality be much closer: 'the study refers to the worst imaginable outcome for amputation (20% mortality and chairbound existence in survivors), whilst at the same time assumes an optimistic 10% operative mortality and 5-year patency' after reconstruction[81]. If even one extra amputation per year is avoided using thrombolysis with t-PA or urokinase, then approximately £30 000 may be saved. This would provide sufficient funding for treatment of 100 patients with t-PA, or 40 patients with urokinase, in preference to streptokinase. The cost of a thrombolytic agent is but a small part of the cost of an admission for acute leg ischaemia.

Clearly further large comparative trials are required to delineate the safest, most efficient agent and method of administration. Only then can data be obtained with which to perform a full cost-benefit analysis.

References

1. Tillett WS and Garner RL. The fibrinolytic activity of haemolytic streptococci. *J Exp Med* 1933; **58**: 485–502

2. Christensen LR and Macleod CM. Proteolytic enzyme of serum; characterisation, activation, and reaction with inhibitors. *J Gen Physiol* 1945; **28**: 559–83

3. Johnson AJ and McCarty WR. The lysis of artificially induced intravascular clots by intravenous infusions of streptokinase. *J Clin Invest* 1959; **38**: 1627–43

4. Koskow DP. Kinetic mechanism of the activation of human plasminogen by streptokinase. *Biochemistry* 1975; **14**: 4459–65

5. Berridge DC, Earnshaw JJ, Westby JC, Makin GS and Hopkinson BR. Fibrinolytic profiles in local low-dose thrombolysis with streptokinase and recombinant tissue plasminogen activator. *Thromb Haemost* 1989; **61**: 275–8

6. Brogden RN, Speight TM and Avery GS. Streptokinase: a review of its clinical pharmacology, mechanism of action and therapeutic uses. *Drugs* 1973; **5**: 357–445

7. Schmutzler R and Koller F. Thrombolytic therapy. In *Poller Recent Advances in Blood Coagulation*. Churchill, London, 1969

8. Elliott JM, Cross DB, Cederhom-Williams S and White HD. Streptokinase titres 1 to 4 years after intravenous streptokinase. *Circulation* 1991; **84**: 11–116

9. Kwaan HC. Hematological aspects of thrombolytic therapy. In Comerota AJ. (ed) *Thrombolytic Therapy*. Grune and Stratton, Orlando, 1988

10. Nora RE and Bell WR. Practical aspects of thrombolytic therapy for deep vein thrombosis. In Comerota AJ (ed) *Thrombolytic Therapy*. Grune and Stratton, Orlando, 1988

11. Kakkar VV, Flanc C, O'Shea M, Flute PT and Clarke MB. Treatment of deep-vein thrombosis with streptokinase. *Br J Surg* 1969; **56**: 178–83

12. Comerota AJ. Complications of thrombolytic therapy. In Comerota AJ. (ed) *Thrombolytic Therapy*. Grune and Stratton, Orlando, 1988

13. Ehrly AM and Lange B. Reduction of blood viscosity and disaggregation of erythrocyte aggregation by streptokinase. In *Theoretical and Clinical Hemorrheology, Proceedings of the International Conference, Heidelberg* 1969. Hartet and Copley, 1971

14. Fitzgerald DJ, Roy L and Fitzgerald GA. Evidence of marked platelet activation following thrombolytic therapy in acute myocardial infarction in man. *Circulation* 1986; **74**: 234

15. Fitzgerald DJ, Roy L, Catella F and Fitzgerald GA. Platelet activation in unstable coronary disease. *N Engl J Med.* 1986; **315**: 983–9

16. Fitzgerald DJ, Catella F, Roy L and Fitzgerald GA. Marked platelet activation *in vivo* after intravenous streptokinase in patients with acute myocardial infarction. *Circulation* 1988; **77**: 142–50

17. Fitzgerald DJ, Roy L, Wright F and Fitzgerald GA. Functional significance of platelet activation following coronary thrombolysis. *Circulation* 1987; **76**: 151

18. MacFarlane RG and Pilling J. Fibrinolytic activity of normal urine. *Nature* 1947; **159**: 779

19. William J. The fibrinolytic activity of urine. *Br J Exp Pathol* 1951; **35**: 530

20. Astrup T and Sterndorff I. Activator of plasminogen in normal urine. *Proc R Soc Med* 1952; **81**: 675–8

21. Bernik MB and Kwaan HC. Plasminogen activator activity in cultures from human tissues. An immunological and histochemical study. *J Clin Invest* 1969; **48**: 1740–53

22. Marzelle J, Combe S, Gigou F and Samama M. Results of thrombolysis in the treatment of arterial ischaemia of the limbs according to mode of administration. *Int Angiol* 1989; **8**: 179–87

23. Cragg AH, Smith TP, Corson JD *et al.* Two urokinase dose regimens in native arterial and graft occlusions: initial results of a prospective, randomised clinical trial. *Radiology* 1991; **178**: 681–6

24. Van Breda A, Katzen BT and Deutsch AS. Urokinase versus streptokinase in local thrombolysis. *Radiology* 1987; **165**: 109–11

25. McNamara TO and Fischer JR. Thrombolysis of peripheral arterial and graft occlusions: improved results using high dose urokinase. *AJR* 1985; **144**: 769–75

26. Nolan C, Hall LS, Barlow GH *et al.* Plasminogen activator from human embryonic kidney cell cultures. *Biochim Biophys Acta* 1977; **496**: 384–400

27. Hussain SS, Gurewich V and Lipinski B. Purification and partial characterisation of a single chain, high molecular weight form of urokinase from human urine. *Arch Biochem Biophys* 1983; **220**: 31–8

28. Collen D, Stassen JM, Blaber M, Winkler M and Verstraete M. Biological and thrombolytic properties of proenzyme and active forms of human urokinase III. Thrombolytic properties of natural and recombinant urokinase in rabbits with experimental jugular vein thrombosis. *Thromb Haemost* 1984; **52**: 27–30

29. Gurewich V, Pannell R, Louie S, Kelley P, Suddith RL and Greenlee R. Effective and fibrin-specific clot lysis by a zymogen precursor form of urokinase (pro-urokinase). A study *in-vitro* and in two animal species. *J Clin Invest* 1984; **73**: 1731–9

30. Gurewich V and Pannell R. Prourokinase – a study of its stability in plasma and of a mechanism for its selective fibrinolytic effect. *Blood* 1986; **67**: 1215–23

31. Zamarron C, Lijnen HR, Van Hoef B and Collen D. Biological and thrombolytic properties of proenzyme and active forms of urokinase. I. Fibrinolytic and fibrinogenolytic properties in human plasma *in vitro* of urokinase obtained from human urine by recombinant DNA technology. *Thromb Haemost* 1984; **52**: 19–23

32. Smith R, Dupe R, English P and Green J. Fibrinolysis with acyl-enzymes: a new approach to thrombolytic therapy. *Nature* 1981; **290**: 505–8

33. Marder VJ, Rothbard RL, Fitzpatrick PG and Francis CW. Rapid lysis of coronary thrombi with anisoylated plasminogen:streptokinase activator complex. *Ann Intern Med* 1986; **104**: 304–10

34. Kasper W, Erbel R, Meinertz T *et al*. Intracoronary thrombolysis with an acylated streptokinase-plasminogen activator (BRL26921) in patients with acute myocardial infarction. *J Am Coll Cardiol* 1984; **2**: 357–63

35. Marder VJ, Francis CW and Norry EC. Dose-ranging study of acylated streptokinase:plasminogen complex (BRL26921). *Thromb Haemost* 1983; **50**: 321

36. Earnshaw JJ, Westby JC, Makin GS and Hopkinson BR. The systemic fibrinolytic effect of BRL26921 during the treatment of acute peripheral arterial occlusions. *Thromb Haemost* 1986; **55**: 259–62

37. Binder BR, Spragg J and Austen KF. Purification and characterisation of human vascular plasminogen activator derived from blood vessel perfusates. *J Biol Chem* 1979; **254**: 1998–2003

38. Rijken DC, Wijngaards G, Zaal-Dejung M *et al*. Purification and partial characterisation of plasminogen activator from human uterine tissue. *Biochem Biophys Acta* 1979; **580**: 140–53

39. Collen D, Rijken DC, Van Damme J and Billiau A. Purification of human tissue-type plasminogen activator in centigram quantities from human melanoma cell culture fluid and its reconditioning for use *in vivo*. *Thromb Haemost* 1982; **48**: 294–6

40. Collen D, Stassen JM, Marafiro B *et al*. Biological properties of human tissue-type plasminogen activator obtained by expression of recombinant DNA in mammalian cells. *J Pharmacol Exp Ther* 1984; **23**: 146–52

41. Pennica D, Holmes WE, Kohn WJ *et al*. Cloning and expression of human tissue plasminogen activator DNA in *E coli*. *Nature* 1983; **301**: 214–21

42. Tran-Chang C, Kruithof EKO and Bachmann F. Tissue-type plasminogen activator increases the binding of Glu-plasminogen to clots. *J Clin Invest* 1984; **74**: 2009–16

43. Lijnen HR and Collen D. Interaction of plasminogen and activators and inhibitors with plasminogen and fibrin. *Semin Thromb Haemostas*. 1982; **8**: 2–10

44. Matsuo O, Rijken DC and Collen D. Comparison of the relative fibrinogenolytic, fibrinolytic and thrombolytic properties of tissue plasminogen activator and urokinase *in vitro*. *Thromb Haemost* 1981; **45**: 225–9

45. Mattson C, Nyberg-Arrhenius V and Wallen P. Dissolution of thrombi by tissue plasminogen activator and streptokinase in an artificial circulating system. *Thromb Res* 1981; **21**: 535–45

46. Wiemer W, Stibbe J, Van Seyen AJ *et al*. Specific lysis of an iliofemoral thrombus by administration of extrinsic (tissue-type) plasminogen activator. *Lancet* 1981; **ii**: 1018–29

47. Berridge DC, Gregson RHS, Westby JC, Hopkinson BR and Makin GS. Randomized trial of intra-arterial recombinant tissue plasminogen activator, intra-venous recombinant tissue plasminogen activator and intra-arterial streptokinase in peripheral arterial thrombolysis. *Br J Surg* 1991; **78**: 988–95

48. Grossbard E (1987) Cited by Sobel BE. Safety and efficacy of tissue-type plasminogen activator produced by recombinant DNA technology. *J Am Coll Cardiol* 1987; **10**: 40B–44B

49. Rabe FE, Becker GJ, Richmond BD *et al.* Contrast extravasation through Dacron grafts: a sequela of low-dose streptokinase therapy. *AJR* 1982; **138**: 917–20

50. Perler BA, Kinnison M and Halden WJ. Transgraft haemorrhage: a serious complication of low-dose thrombolytic therapy. *J Vasc Surg* 1986; **3**: 936–83

51. Marder VJ, Donahoe JF, Bell WJ *et al.* Changes in the plasminogen-plasmin fibrinolytic system during urokinase therapy: comparison of tissue culture urokinase with urinary source urokinase in patients with pulmonary embolism. *J Lab Clin Med* 1978; **92**: 721–9

52. Martin M. Thrombolytic therapy in arterial thromboembolism. *Prog Cardiovasc Dis* 1979; **21**: 351–74

53. van de Werf F, Ludbrook PA, Bergman SR *et al.* Coronary thrombolysis with tissue type plasminogen activator in patients with evolving myocardial infarction. *N Engl J Med* 1984; **310**: 609–13

54. Collen D. Tissue-type plasminogen activator: therapeutic potential in thrombotic disease states. *Drugs* 1986; **31**: 1–5

55. Collen D, Stassen J-M, Stump DC and Verstraete M. Synergism of thrombolytic agents *in vivo*. *Circulation* 1986, **74**: 838–42

56. Collen D, Stump DC and Van de Werf F. Coronary thrombolysis in patients with acute myocardial infarction by intravenous infusion of synergistic thrombolytic agents. *Am Heart J* 1986; **112**: 1083–4

57. Graor RA, Risius B, Denny KM *et al.* Local thrombolysis in the treatment of thrombosed arteries, bypass grafts, and arteriovenous fistulas. *J Vasc Surg* 1985; **2**: 406–14

58. Earnshaw JJ, Westby JC, Makin GS and Hopkinson BR. Local thrombolytic therapy of acute peripheral arterial ischaemia with tissue plasminogen activator: a dose ranging study. *Br J Surg* 1988; **75**: 1196–1200

59. The TIMI study group. The thrombolysis in myocardial infarction (TIMI) trial. Phase I findings. *N Engl J Med* 1985; **312**: 932–6

60. Verstraete M, Bory M, Collen D *et al.* Randomised trial of intravenous recombinant tissue-type plasminogen activator versus intravenous streptokinase in acute myocardial infarction. Report from the European Cooperative Study Group for Recombinant Tissue-type Plasminogen Activator. *Lancet* 1985; **ii**: 842–7

61. Wilcox RG, von der Lippe G, Olsson OG *et al.* Trial of tissue plasminogen activator for mortality reduction in acute myocardial infarction. Anglo-Scandinavian study of early thrombolysis (ASSET). *Lancet* 1988; **11**: 525–30

62. Gardiner GA, Harrington DP, Koltun W *et al.* Salvage of occluded arterial bypass grafts by means of thrombolysis. *J Vasc Surg* 1989; **9**: 426–31

63. Walker WJ and Giddings AEB. A protocol for the safe treatment of acute lower limb ischaemia with intra-arterial streptokinase and surgery. *Br J Surg* 1988; **75**: 1189–92

64. Mori KW, Bookstein JJ, Heeny DJ *et al.* Selective streptokinase infusion: clinical and laboratory correlates. *Radiology* 1983; **148**: 677–82

65. Risius B, Graor RA, Geisinger MA *et al.* Thrombolytic therapy with recombinant human tissue-type plasminogen activator: a comparison of two doses. *Radiology* 1987; **164**: 465–8

66. Verstraete M, Hess H, Mahler A *et al.* Femoro-popliteal artery thrombolysis with intra-arterial infusion of recombinant tissue-type plasminogen activator – report of a pilot trial. *Eur J Vasc Surg* 1988; **3**: 155–9

67. Lonsdale RJ, Berridge DC, Earnshaw JJ *et al.* Recombinant tissue-type plasminogen activator is superior to streptokinase for local intra-arterial thrombolysis. *Br J Surg* 1992; **79**: 272–5

68. Earnshaw JJ, Scott DJA, Horrocks M and Baird RN. Choice of agent for peripheral thrombolysis. *Br J Surg* 1993; **80**: 25–7

69. Berridge DC, Makin GS and Hopkinson BR. Local low-dose thrombolytic therapy: the risk of stroke or major haemorrhage. *Br J Surg* 1989; **76**: 1230–33

70. Loscalzo J and Vaughan DE. Tissue plasminogen activator promotes platelet disaggregation in plasma. *J Clin Invest* 1987; **79**: 1749–55
71. Becker RC. Recombinant t-PA and platelet activity. *Cleveland Clin J Med* 1990; **57**: 537–41
72. Meyerovitz MF, Goldhaber SZ, Reagan K *et al.* Recombinant tissue-type plasminogen activator versus urokinase in peripheral arterial and graft occlusions: a randomised trial. *Radiology* 1990: **175**: 75–8
73. Cheshire NJW, Wolfe JHN, Noone MA, Davies L and Drummond M. The economics of femorocrural reconstruction for critical leg ischemia with and without autologous vein. *J Vasc Surg* 1992; **15**: 167–75
74. Hess H, Ingrisch H, Mietaschk A and Rath H. Local low dose thrombolytic therapy of peripheral arterial occlusions. *N Engl Med* 1982; **307**: 1627–30
75. Lammer J, Pilger E, Neumayer K and Schreyer H. Intra-arterial fibrinolysis: long term results. *Radiology* 1985; **154**: 75–7
76. Browse DJ, Barr H, Torrie EPH and Galland RB. Limitations to the widespread usage of low-dose intra-arterial thrombolysis. *Eur J Vasc Surg* 1991; **5**: 445–9
77. Dacey LJ, Dow RW, McDaniel MD *et al.* Cost-effectiveness of intra-arterial thrombolytic therapy. *Arch Surg* 1988; **123**: 1218–23
78. Graor RA, Risius B, Young JR *et al.* Thrombolysis of peripheral arterial bypass grafts: surgical thrombectomy compared with thrombolysis. *J Vasc Surg* 1988; **7**: 347–55
79. Janosik JE, Bettman MA, Kaul AF and Souney PF. Therapeutic alternatives for subacute peripheral arterial occlusion. Comparison by outcome, length of stay, and hospital charges. *Invest Radiol* 1991; **26**: 921–5
80. Allen DR, Fergus MEB and Chant ADB. Cost effectiveness of treating critical ischaemia using quality adjusted life years. *Br J Surg* 1990; **77**: A348
81. Fyfe NCM. Assessment of the rehabilitation of amputees. *Curr Prac Surg* 1992; **4**: 90–8

Chapter 9

Adjuvant drugs for peripheral thrombolysis

R. J. Lonsdale

Introduction

Adjuvant therapy has a potential role in peripheral thrombolysis in three areas: during lysis, during angioplasty at completion of thrombolysis and after lysis. Adjuvant therapy given during thrombolysis may improve the efficacy of the thrombolytic agent. This may have two beneficial effects: the rate of lysis may be increased, resulting in shorter treatment times, and the proportion of patients being successfully lysed may be optimized. Alternatively, adjuvant therapy may be given during lysis in an attempt to reduce the incidence of side-effects such as peri-catheter thrombosis. Should angioplasty be required on completion of lysis, adjuvant agents may reduce the incidence of complications. Finally, adjuvant therapy after lysis may have a role in reducing the incidence of subsequent re-thrombosis and hence improve long-term patency rates.

Four groups of drugs have been investigated as adjuvant therapy to thrombolytic agents – anti-platelet agents, anti-coagulants, vasodilators and synergistic thrombolytic agents which were considered previously in Chapter 8 (Table 9.1). The use of these agents varies widely from centre to centre

Table 9.1 Anticipated benefits of adjuvant agents advocated for peripheral thrombolysis

	During lysis	*During angioplasty*	*After lysis*
Anti-platelet agents	Enhanced lytic effect	Prevention of immediate re-thrombosis	Prevention of late re-occlusion
Anti-coagulants	Reduced pericatheter thrombosis	Prevention of immediate re-thrombosis	Prevention of late re-occlusion
Vasodilators	Decrease vasoconstriction	Prevention of immediate re-thrombosis	
Synergistic thrombolytic agents	Enhanced lytic effect		

and as yet no clinical trial has established a definite role for any single adjuvant agent in peripheral thrombolysis. This may in part be due to the small number of published comparative studies in peripheral thrombolysis. This deficiency means that clinical decisions about the use of adjuvant therapy in peripheral thrombolysis must often be based on the extrapolation of findings in experimental studies or studies of coronary thrombolysis. In this chapter the rationale for the use of adjuvant agents in peripheral thrombolysis and the available experimental and clinical data are reviewed.

Anti-platelet therapy during thrombolysis

RATIONALE

The fundamental role of platelet activation and aggregation in the formation of arterial thrombi has been established for over 100 years[1]. The role that platelets play during the lysis of arterial thrombi is less well understood. There is, however, evidence suggesting that platelet activation occurs during thrombolytic therapy, that this platelet activation may cause resistance to the thrombolytic therapy and that the use of an anti-platelet agent may be beneficial.

The evidence that platelet activation occurs during thrombolysis stems from a number of studies in which an increase in products of platelet activation, such as the metabolites of thromboxane A_2 or the platelet-specific protein beta thromboglobulin, has been documented during coronary thrombolysis in man and in animal models[2-5]. Following infusion of thrombolytic agents platelets become more responsive to aggregating agents[6], platelet survival is shortened[7,8] and bleeding time increased[9,10]. *In vitro* evidence suggests that, particularly with streptokinase, this platelet activation is the result of a direct effect of the thrombolytic agent itself[2,11-13].

Platelet function in patients with peripheral arterial thromboses undergoing thrombolysis has been investigated in one study[14]. It was found that plasma beta thromboglobulin levels were increased during lysis with intra-arterial streptokinase but there was no other evidence of platelet activation. After lysis, platelet responsiveness to aggrega-ting agents was increased, possibly as a result of heparin administration[15].

The evidence that platelet activation results in resistance to thrombolysis arises from the observation that 20% of coronary artery occlusions fail to re-perfuse and that these resistant thrombi are, in some cases, particularly rich in platelets[16].

EXPERIMENTAL STUDIES

Clear evidence has been obtained in a variety of experimental settings that anti-platelet therapy enhances the effects of thrombolytic agents (Table 9.2). *In vitro*, Terres *et al.*[17] found that prostaglandin PGE_1, but not aspirin, enhanced thrombolysis of platelet and fibrin thrombi by urokinase. In animal models of coronary artery thrombosis, aspirin[18], sulotroban (a specific thromboxane A_2 receptor antagonist)[19], monoclonal anti-platelet antibody[3,20] and poly-peptide platelet glycoprotein IIb/IIIa receptor antagonists[21] have all been shown to enhance thrombolysis. Only one similar study has been reported investigating the role of anti-platelet agents in

Table 9.2 Experimental evidence supporting the use of anti-platelet agents during thrombolysis

Anti-platelet agent	Thrombolytic agent	Study group	Effect	Reference
PGE$_1$	Urokinase	In vitro	Faster lysis	Terres 1989[17]
Aspirin	t-PA	Dog coronary artery thrombosis	Faster lysis	Haskel 1991[18]
Sulotroban	t-PA	Dog coronary artery thrombosis	Faster lysis Re-occlusion rate reduced	Shebuski 1988[19]
Monoclonal anti-platelet antibody	t-PA	Dog coronary artery thrombosis	Higher rate of reperfusion	Gold 1988[20]
Polypeptide platelet receptor antagonist	t-PA	Dog coronary artery thrombosis	Faster lysis Re-occlusion rate reduced	Yasuda 1991[21]
PGE$_1$	t-PA	Feline femoral artery thrombosis	Faster lysis	Humphrey 1991[22]

thrombolysis in an animal model of peripheral arterial thrombosis. Humphrey and Schaub[22] reported that the combination of prostaglandin E$_1$ 0.3 g/kg/min with intravenous t-PA shortened the time to reperfusion when compared to t-PA alone.

CLINICAL STUDIES

The clearest evidence of the benefit of adjuvant anti-platelet agents during thrombolysis was obtained in the ISIS-2 study[23], in which the addition of aspirin (160 mg/day for 1 month) to streptokinase (1.5 million u) in the treatment of acute myocardial infarction reduced the 5-week vascular mortality from 10.4% to 8.0% without an increase in the incidence of major haemorrhage. Some of the benefit of aspirin is probably due to prevention of coronary artery re-occlusion after successful recanalization. However, it almost certainly also plays a role in reducing the time taken to achieve recanalization, thereby limiting myocardial damage.

There are few studies of anti-platelet therapy during peripheral thrombolysis. In one large series, aspirin 500 mg twice or three times daily was given to all patients beginning the day prior to thrombolysis[24,25]. This combination appeared not to be associated with an increased incidence of haemorrhagic complications, though there was no control group, so it is impossible to assess the actual benefit of adjuvant aspirin. Furthermore, in this study the infusion regimen allowed a maximum duration of only 3 hours. Some caution is therefore needed in extrapolating this experience to thrombolysis in the UK where infusions are often continued for over 24 hours.

The prolonged action of aspirin has led to fears that, should bleeding occur, it would be more difficult to control because of persisting inhibition of platelet function. In view of this the three comparative studies of adjuvant

Table 9.3 Clinical trials of adjuvant anti-platelet agents in thrombolysis

Anti-platelet agent	Thrombolytic agent	Study group	Patients studied (no.)	Effect	Reference
Aspirin	Streptokinase	Acute myocardial infarction	8592	Reduced 35-day vascular mortality	ISIS-2[23]
Sulotroban	Streptokinase	Peripheral lysis	21	Faster lysis, increased bleeding	Lonsdale[14]
Iloprost	t-PA	Peripheral lysis	32	No beneficial effect	Lonsdale[26]

anti-platelet therapy during peripheral thrombolysis used short-acting agents (Table 9.3). The largest such study was conducted using the short-acting thromboxane A_2 antagonist, sulotroban, which was compared to placebo in a multicentre trial of approximately 80 patients. This study was stopped prior to completion and the results not reported. An interim analysis (presented at Daltroban Consultative Meeting, Frankfurt, October 1990) suggested little difference between patients receiving sulotroban and those receiving placebo with regard to successful lysis and the duration of infusion required to achieve lysis. A smaller single-centre study examined a range of doses of sulotroban in comparison to placebo as adjuvant therapy in patients receiving low-dose local streptokinase[14]. In this study sulotroban did not increase the proportion of patients successfully lysed but it appeared to reduce the time taken to achieve lysis. The median time to lysis was 25.5 hours in patients randomized to adjuvant sulotroban and 48.5 hours in patients randomized to placebo. However, at the highest dose of sulotroban tested (8 mg/min), there was an excess of major haemorrhagic complications.

In both studies using sulotroban the anti-platelet agent was given systemically. Since the primary intention of giving adjuvant anti-platelet therapy during lysis is to inhibit platelet activation at the site of the thrombus rather than to inhibit systemic platelet function, this route of administration may have been inappropriate. Therefore, in a third study adjuvant anti-platelet therapy was given with the thrombolytic agent via the intra-arterial catheter in a double-blind randomized trial[26]. The agent used in this case was iloprost, a synthetic prostanoid (Schering), and the thrombolytic agent was t-PA. The results were disappointing: adding iloprost did not reduce the lysis time compared to placebo or increase the number of patients with successful lysis. This route of administration did at least appear to be safe: there was only one major bleed in 16 patients who received the combined treatment.

In summary, although there is a sound rationale for using anti-platelet therapy during peripheral thrombolysis, particularly when the thrombolytic agent used is streptokinase, and although adjuvant anti-platelet therapy is of proven benefit during coronary thrombolysis, there are no clinical studies supporting its use in peripheral thrombolysis. The studies that have been reported do not exclude a possible benefit from anti-platelet therapy but it is clear that if such a benefit exists it is likely to be small. The role of aspirin remains uncertain prior to or during thrombolysis. Furthermore, it is clear that studies investigating the potential use of adjuvant anti-platelet therapy need to be conducted with caution because of the possible risk of haemorrhage.

Anti-coagulation during peripheral thrombolysis

RATIONALE

The argument for using heparin or thrombin inhibitors during peripheral thrombolysis is that it reduces the incidence of pericatheter thrombosis. This has been reported in up to 26% of patients[27] and may exacerbate the limb ischaemia. Although it is usually possible to clear peri-catheter thrombus by withdrawing the arterial catheter proximally and perfusing the peri-catheter thrombus with lytic agent, this is not always the case and persisting peri-catheter thrombus may contribute to the failure of lysis.

In intravenous coronary thrombolysis it is thought that heparin is of value by potentiating the effect of thrombolytic agents, in particular t-PA. Recent evidence demonstrated that thrombin activity is increased in some patients with acute myocardial infarction[28] and that markers of heightened thrombin activity may identify patients who risk unsuccessful reperfusion[29]. In this respect the rationale for the use of heparin or thrombin antagonists during thrombolysis is very similar to the rationale for anti-platelet agents.

EXPERIMENTAL EVIDENCE

Prevention of peri-catheter thrombosis by anti-thrombotic agents has not been examined experimentally and deserves attention. A number of studies have examined the use of heparin and hirudin to potentiate the effects of thrombolytic agents. The results of these studies have not been conclusive, with some demonstrating a beneficial effect of heparin[30,31], whilst others demonstrate no advantage[32].

CLINICAL PRACTICE

The first reported study assessed the value of heparin with t-PA for coronary thrombolysis in achieving early (90 minutes) coronary artery patency[33]. In this study the addition of heparin did not improve the efficacy of t-PA. A number of other studies, although by no means all, have shown that heparin improves late patency rates. This may reflect a role for heparin in preventing re-thrombosis after lysis rather than an advantage during lysis itself[34]. In the largest study of thrombolysis for myocardial infarction (ISIS-3) no major benefit was demonstrated for the addition of heparin to the thrombolytic regimen[35].

In peripheral thrombolysis there appears to be an even distribution between those centres using adjuvant heparin[36-39] and those not[40-42]. Three non-randomized comparative studies[43-45] have examined the effect of heparin on the results of peripheral thrombolysis and have not demonstrated any advantage. In each case, the number of patients studied was small.

The main risk of adjuvant heparin during thrombolysis is haemorrhage. Both streptokinase and, to a lesser extent, t-PA have a direct anti-coagulant effect, particularly after prolonged administration. Injudicious routine heparin administration may further prolong coagulation times and thereby increase the risk of haemorrhagic complications.

Considering the lack of firm evidence of benefit from heparin during peripheral thrombolysis, it is difficult to give sensible advice on its use. A balanced view might be that heparin does not appear to enhance the efficacy of thrombolytic agents, that systemic administration to prevent peri-catheter thrombosis risks an increase in haemorrhagic complications but that local administration to prevent peri-catheter thrombosis may be appropriate. Such local administration should be considered in the light of the catheter placement. Instillation of heparin via an arterial sheath so that it washes over a coaxially placed catheter, or administration down an arterial catheter wedged into the top of an arterial thrombus, are both likely to result in a local anti-coagulant effect around the arterial catheter with less systemic effect. Administration of heparin via an arterial catheter placed so that its tip lies in the distal portion of thrombus will result in heparin being delivered to the run-off vessels rather than around the catheter and can be expected to have little effect on the incidence of peri-catheter thrombosis.

Vasodilators during peripheral thrombolysis

RATIONALE

Continuing platelet deposition has been demonstrated in patients suffering lower limb arterial thromboses up to 28 days after the onset of symptoms[46]. This is presumed to be the result of ongoing platelet activation. Potent vasoconstrictors such as thromboxane A_2 and serotonin released as a result of platelet activation at the distal margin of the thrombus may wash out into the run-off vessels and exacerbate the degree of ischaemia. If significant vasoconstriction occurs, limb blood flow may be reduced leading to stasis and propagation of thrombus. Since, as seen above, the administration of thrombolytic agents results in the release of thromboxane A_2 metabolites there is a rationale for giving vasodilator agents concurrently with thrombolytic agents in an attempt to prevent vasoconstriction.

EXPERIMENTAL STUDIES

Experimental evidence suggesting that vasodilator drugs may be of benefit in thrombolysis comes from studies investigating agents with both vasodilator and anti-platelet actions. Prostacyclin, prostaglandin E_1 and the thromboxane receptor antagonists fall into this category. It is difficult to distinguish whether the vasodilator or platelet inhibitory properties of these drugs are more important. Such a distinction is probably irrelevant since platelet-derived agents are largely responsible for vasoconstriction and therefore platelet inhibition itself has an indirect vasodilator effect. Drugs such as nitrates that were regarded primarily as vasodilators have, since the discovery of endothelium-derived relaxing factor (nitric oxide)[47], been recognized also to have anti-platelet properties.

CLINICAL STUDIES

Clinical studies of anti-platelet agents with vasodilator properties have been described previously, and failed to demonstrate any benefit. None of the major series of patients treated with peripheral thrombolysis have included vasodilator drugs as part of the thrombolytic regimen. Their use has, however, been recommended in at least one review[48].

Synergistic infusions of thrombolytic agents

Synergism between thrombolytic agents with different modes of action has been confirmed both experimentally[49,50] and clinically[51-53] as described in Chapter 8. The significance of this finding for peripheral thrombolysis has yet to be determined.

Adjuvant agents during angioplasty

In almost all centres practising peripheral thrombolysis, immediate angioplasty of any underlying stenosis is recommended on completion of lysis. Although there are no controlled trials to justify this approach most clinicians believe that delay in performing angioplasty risks re-thrombosis of the treated arterial segment. The angioplasty technique in this situation is the same as that routinely used and therefore adjuvant therapies used during routine angioplasty are applicable. In contrast, angioplasty is not routinely performed immediately after coronary thrombolysis since it is believed the risk of re-thrombosis is smaller if angioplasty is delayed. There are also logistical problems with the large number of coronary patients who would require cardiac catheterization. Therefore, in coronary thrombolysis there is no analogous situation from which we can extrapolate the findings of research to peripheral thrombolysis.

Anti-platelet therapy during angioplasty

RATIONALE

Routine angioplasty is complicated by early re-thrombosis in between 1% and 7% of cases[54]. A similar incidence of early re-thrombosis has been reported following peripheral thrombolysis[55], although the re-thrombosis rate in patients having completion angioplasty is not usually reported separately from patients not having angioplasty. Platelet activation at the site of the angioplasty has been implicated in this early re-thrombosis[56]. Angioplasty results in splitting of the arterial intima with exposure of underlying media[57]. Platelets may adhere to the subendothelial structures, become activated and aggregate resulting in thrombus formation. Inhibition of this process would appear to be desirable.

CLINICAL STUDIES

Most studies assessing the role of anti-platelet therapy (usually aspirin) as an adjuvant to angioplasty began treatment after the procedure and have assessed its efficacy in preventing late re-thrombosis. No study assessed the efficacy of aspirin or other anti-platelet drugs in preventing early re-thrombosis. Given the comparative rarity of early re-thrombosis such studies would need to be very large. Some investigators have attempted to circumvent this requirement for large numbers by dispensing with clinical end points and examining platelet deposition assessed by radioisotope techniques[58,59]. These studies suffer from the drawback that they assume a direct, causal link between platelet deposition and clinical re-thrombosis. However, if this is accepted then these studies suggest that anti-platelet agents reduce platelet deposition and are beneficial in preventing early re-thrombosis after angioplasty. It is worth pointing out that many centres do not use aspirin prior to angioplasty, or anticoagulants, and yet still report excellent results[60].

Before directly extrapolating the practice in routine angioplasty to angioplasty after lysis, a little caution needs to be exercised. This is particularly because some patients undergoing lysis, particularly with streptokinase, suffer a marked hypofibrinogenaemia[61] which, in combination with profound platelet inhibition, is associated with an increased incidence of bleeding[26]. It seems sensible to advise that plasma fibrinogen levels are checked and aspirin deferred in patients suffering hypofibrinoginaemia. On balance, because aspirin has a prolonged action it may be better to avoid its use at this time. New shorter acting anti-platelet agents may in the future prove to be useful.

Anti-coagulation and vasodilators during completion angioplasty

RATIONALE

The potential exists for thrombin formation and hence re-thrombosis at an angioplasty site because of activation of the extrinsic coagulation pathway by subendothelial tissue factor. Spasm, particularly in distal arteries, induced by the intra-lumenal passage of arterial catheters may exacerbate this process. Clearly it is desirable to avoid this complication and anti-coagulation and/or the administration of vasodilators may be appropriate.

CLINICAL PRACTICE

Heparin is almost uniformly used during routine angioplasty and indeed was advocated by Dotter and Judkins in their first paper[62]. The recommended dose is 5000 u given via the arterial catheter before balloon inflation.

A number of vasodilators are available for the treatment of spasm: lignocaine 50 mg, tolazoline 25 mg and more recently nitroglycerine 100 μg boluses up to a maximum of 500 μg. These are all usually given via the arterial catheter. An alternative is sublingual nifedipine 10–20 mg. In some centres vasodilators are routinely given as prophylaxis against arterial spasm but the majority appear to reserve their use for the treatment of spasm when it occurs.

This policy of routine intra-arterial heparin with vasodilator administration when spasm is encountered during angioplasty after thrombolysis is probably reasonable. Heparin should be omitted or reduced in those patients with prolonged coagulation times as a result of thrombolytic therapy.

Adjuvant therapy after thrombolysis

Prevention of re-thrombosis following vascular intervention remains another area in which there are few proven facts. Anti-platelet therapy is of definite benefit in reducing the incidence of re-occlusion in patients with synthetic vascular grafts[63,64]. Its value or indeed the value of oral anti-coagulants in reducing re-occlusion rates in vein grafts has not been proved, although the evidence suggests that both reduce late mortality in vascular patients[65,66]. Similarly, there is little data demonstrating the value of anti-platelet or oral anti-coagulant therapy following peripheral angioplasty.

In acute myocardial infarction anti-platelet therapy, usually with low-dose aspirin, is routinely given to all patients in whom no contraindication exists whether or not they have been treated with thrombolysis. In these patients it has a beneficial effect on both short- and long-term mortality[23,67]. After successful coronary thrombolysis, studies have demonstrated a beneficial effect of anti-platelet agents in preventing re-occlusion[18–21,68].

Only a handful of studies have reported long-term results following peripheral thrombolysis and none in which the value of anti-platelet or anti-coagulant therapy has been assessed. The long-term results of three of the largest series[24,69–71] are remarkably similar if an allowance is made for the exclusion of a poor prognostic group (those without angiographically demonstrable run off) in one of the series[69]. The policy for adjuvant therapy after lysis varied between these units. Hess et al. used aspirin and dipyridamole in most patients; only patients who had embolic occlusions received oral anti-coagulants. Lammer et al., by contrast, anti-coagulated all patients following thrombolysis. In Nottingham, the policy was a minimum of 6 months oral anti-coagulation with warfarin followed by low-dose aspirin. In the series in which poorer late results were reported[71] (50% patency at 1 year following successful lysis in contrast to about 80% patency in the other centres), patients did not receive either oral anti-coagulation or aspirin. The evidence would suggest that prophylaxis against re-occlusion should be given following thrombolysis but that it makes little difference whether this consists of low-dose aspirin or oral anti-coagulation with warfarin.

Summary

The use of adjuvant therapy in peripheral thrombolysis has not been shown in clinical trials to be of benefit. The theoretical benefits accruing from adjuvant therapy must be weighed against a possible increased risk of bleeding.

In view of this lack of clinical evidence, guidelines for the use of adjuvant therapy are bound to be somewhat arbitrary. Nevertheless a reasonable policy would be to avoid adjuvant agents during thrombolysis, to give heparin and vasodilators if required during completion angioplasty and aspirin or warfarin for long-term prevention of re-thrombosis. When an arterial sheath is used for thrombolysis with a catheter passed coaxially through it, a low dose of heparin (e.g. 250 u/h) may be infused through the sheath to avoid peri-catheter thrombosis, but this may not be better than simply dividing the dose of thrombolytic agent infused between the catheter and the sheath.

The dose of intra-arterial heparin given during angioplasty should be modified or omitted in patients whose coagulation times are prolonged as a result of the thrombolytic therapy, but in patients with normal coagulation a bolus dose of 3000 u would be appropriate. It would seem sensible to avoid aspirin or warfarin during the first 48 hours after thrombolysis since both have a prolonged action and, should re-thrombosis occur during this critical period, may interfere with the recommencement of lysis. Therefore intravenous heparin should be given for at least 48 hours, starting when the thrombin clotting time is shorter than 60 seconds. The dose of heparin should be adjusted to maintain the activated partial thromboplastin time at approximately twice normal until the patient is established on warfarin or until aspirin is commenced.

References

1. Bizzozero J. Ueber einen neuen Formbestand des Blutes und dessen Rolle bei der Thrombose und der Blutgerinnung. *Virch Arch* 1882; **90**: 261–332
2. Fitzgerald DJ, Catella F, Roy L and FitzGerald GA. Marked platelet activation *in vivo* after intravenous streptokinase in patients with acute myocardial infarction. *Circulation* 1988; **77**; 142–50
3. Fitzgerald DJ, Wright F and FitzGerald GA. Increased thromboxane biosynthesis during coronary thrombolysis. Evidence that platelet activation and thromboxane A_2 modulate the response to tissue-type plasminogen activator *in vivo*. *Circ Res* 1989; **65**; 83–94
4. Fitzgerald DJ and FitzGerald GA. Role of thrombin and thromboxane A_2 in reocclusion following coronary thrombolysis with tissue-type plasminogen activator. *Proc Natl Acad Sci USA* 1989; **86**: 7585–9
5. Kerins DM, Roy L, FitzGerald GA and Fitzgerald DJ. Platelet and vascular function during coronary thrombolysis with tissue-type plasminogen activator. *Circulation* 1989; **80**: 1718–25
6. Ohlstein EH, Storer B, Fujita T and Shebuski RJ. Tissue-type plasminogen activator and streptokinase induce platelet hyperaggregability in the rabbit. *Throm Res* 1987; **46**: 575–85
7. Greenberg JP, Packham MA, Guccione MA, Rand ML, Reimers H-J and Mustard JF. Survival of rabbit platelets treated *in vitro* with chymotrypsin, plasmin, trypsin or neuraminidase. *Blood* 1979; **53**: 916–27
8. Winocour PD, Kinlough-Rathbone RL, Richardson M and Mustard JF. Reversal of shortened platelet survival in rats by the antifibrinolytic agent, epsilon aminocaproic acid. *J Clin Invest* 1983; **71**: 159–64
9. Kowalski E, Budzynski AZ, Kopec M, Latallo ZS, Lipinski B and Wegryznowicz Z. Studies on the molecular pathology and pathogenesis of bleeding in severe fibrinolytic states in dogs. *Throm Diath Haemorrh* 1964; **12**: 69–85
10. Gimple LW, Gold HK, Leinbach RC *et al.* Correlation between template bleeding times and spontaneous bleeding during treatment of acute myocardial infarction with recombinant tissue-type plasminogen activator. *Circulation* 1989; **80**: 581–8
11. Heptinstall S, Berridge DC and Judge H. Effects of streptokinase and recombinant tissue plasminogen activator on platelet aggregation in whole blood. *Platelets* 1990; **1**: 177–88
12. Berridge DC, Burgess-Wilson ME, Westby JC, Hopkinson BR and Makin GS. Differential effects of low-dose tissue plasminogen activator and streptokinase on platelet aggregation. *Br J Surg* 1989; **76**: 1026–30
13. Vaughan DE, Van Houtte, E, Declerck PJ and Collen D. Streptokinase-induced platelet aggregation. Prevalence and mechanism. *Circulation* 1991; **84**: 84–91
14. Lonsdale RJ, Heptinstall S, Westby JC, Berridge DC, Wenham PW, Hopkinson BR and Makin GS. A study of the use of the thromboxane A_2 antagonist sulotroban, in combination with streptokinase for local thrombolysis in patients with recent peripheral

arterial occlusions: clinical effects, platelet function and fibrinolytic parameters. *Thromb Haemost* 1993; **69**: 103–11

15. Mikhailidis DP, Barradas MA, O'Donoghue S and Dandona P. Evidence for *in vivo* platelet activation following the injection of conventional unfractionated heparin. *Platelets* 1990; **1**: 189–92

16. Jang I-K, Gold HK, Ziskind AA *et al*. Differential sensitivity of erythrocyte-rich and platelet-rich arterial thrombi to lysis with recombinant tissue-type plasminogen activator. A possible explanation for resistance to coronary thrombolysis. *Circulation* 1989; **79**: 920–8

17. Terres W, Beythien, C, Kupper W and Bleifeld W. Effects of aspirin and prostaglandin E_1 on *in vitro* thrombolysis with urokinase. Evidence for a possible role of inhibiting platelet activity in thrombolysis. *Circulation* 1989; **79**: 1309–14

18. Haskel EJ, Prager NA, Sobel BE, Abendschein DR. Relative efficacy of antithrombin compared with antiplatelet agents in accelerating coronary thrombolysis and preventing early reocclusion. *Circulation* 1991; **83**: 1048–56

19. Shebuski RJ, Smith JM, Storer BL, Granett JR and Bugelski PJ. Influence of selective endoperoxide/thromboxane A_2 receptor antagonism with sulotroban on lysis time and reocclusion rate after tissue plasminogen activator-induced coronary thrombolysis in the dog. *J Pharmacol Exp Ther* 1988; **246**: 790–796

20. Gold HK, Coller BS, Yasuda T *et al*. Rapid and sustained coronary artery recanalization with combined bolus injection of recombinant tissue-type plasminogen activator and monoclonal antiplatelet GPIIb/IIIa antibody in a canine preparation. *Circulation* 1988; **77**: 670–7

21. Yasuda, T, Gold HK, Leinbach RC *et al*. Kistrin, a polypeptide platelet GPIIb/IIIa receptor antagonist, enhances and sustains coronary arterial thrombolysis with recombinant tissue-type plasminogen activator in a canine preparation. *Circulation* 1991; **83**: 1038–47

22. Humphrey WR and Schaub RG. Effect of intravenous prostaglandin E_1 on thrombolysis induced by human recombinant tissue-type plasminogen activator in feline peripheral arterial thrombosis. *Fibrinolysis* 1991; **5**: 71–9

23. ISIS-2 (Second International Study of Infarct Survival) Collaborative Group. Randomised trial of intravenous streptokinase, oral aspirin, both, or neither among 17 187 cases of suspected acute myocardial infarction. *Lancet* 1988; **ii**: 349–60

24. Hess H, Mietaschk A and Bruckl R. Peripheral arterial occlusions: a 6-year experience with local low-dose thrombolytic therapy. *Radiology* 1987; **163**: 753–8

25. Hess H. Thrombolytic therapy in peripheral vascular disease. *Br J Surg* 1990; **77**: 1083–4

26. Lonsdale RJ, Astill JY, Whitaker SC *et al*. Adjuvant iloprost does not improve results of local thrombolysis with recombinant tissue plasminogen activator. *Br J Surg* 1993; **80**: A656

27. Eskridge JM, Becker GJ, Rabe FE *et al*. Catheter-related thrombosis and fibrinolytic therapy. *Radiology* 1983; **149**: 429–432

28. Eisenberg PR, Sherman LA, Schectman K, Perez J, Sobel BE and Jaffe AS. Fibrinopeptide A: a marker of acute coronary thrombosis. *Circulation* 1985; **71**: 912–8

29. Gulba DC, Barthels M, Westhoff-Bleck M *et al*. Increased thrombin levels during thrombolytic therapy in acute myocardial infarction. Relevance for the success of therapy. *Circulation* 1991; **83**: 937–44

30. Cercek B, Lew AS, Hod H, Yano J, Reddy NKN and Ganz W. Enhancement of thrombolysis with tissue-type plasminogen activator by pretreatment with heparin. *Circulation* 1986; **74**: 583–7

31. Mickelson JK, Simpson PJ and Lucchesi BR. Effects of heparin and intravenous tissue plasminogen activator or streptokinase in a canine model of coronary artery thrombosis (Abstr). *Clin Res* 1987; **35**: 305

32. Agnelli G, Pascucci C, Cosmi B and Nenci GG. Effects of therapeutic doses of heparin on thrombolysis with tissue-type plasminogen activator in rabbits. *Blood* 1990; **76**: 2030–6

33. Topol EJ, George BS, Kereiakes DJ *et al*. A randomized controlled trial of intravenous tissue plasminogen activator and early intravenous heparin in acute myocardinal infarction. *Circulation* 1989; **79**: 281–6

34. Prins MH and Hirsh J. Heparin as an adjunctive treatment after thrombolytic therapy for acute myocardial infarction *Am J Cardiol* 1991; **67**: 3A–11A
35. ISIS-3 (Third International Study of Infarct Survival Collaborative Group). A randomised comparison of streptokinase vs tissue plasminogen activator vs anistreplase and of aspirin plus heparin vs aspirin alone among 41 299 cases of suspected myocardial infarction. *Lancet* 1992; **339**: 753–70
36. Verstraete M, Hess H, Mahler F *et al*. Femoro-popliteal artery thrombolysis with intra-arterial infusion of recombinant tissue-type plasminogen activator – report of a pilot trial. *Eur J Vasc Surg* 1988; **2**: 155–9
37. Dawson KJ, Reddy K, Platts AD and Hamilton G. Results of a recently instituted programme of thrombolytic therapy in acute lower limb ischaemia. *Br J Surg* 1991; **78**: 409–11
38. Barr H, Lancashire MJR, Torrie EPH, Galland RB. Intra-arterial thrombolytic therapy in the management of acute and chronic limb ischaemia. *Br J Surg* 1991; **76**: 284–7
39. McNamara TO, Bomberger RA and Merchant RF. Intra-arterial urokinase as the initial therapy for acutely ischaemic lower limbs. *Circulation* 1991; **83**(suppl. I): 106–119
40. Graor RA, Risius B, Young JR *et al*. Low-dose streptokinase for selective thrombolysis: systemic effects and complications. *Radiology* 1984; **152**: 35–9
41. Risius B, Graor RA, Geisinger MA, Zelch MG, Lucas FV and Young JR. Thrombolytic therapy with recombinant human tissue-type plasminogen activator: a comparison of two doses. *Radiology* 1987; **164**: 465–8
42. Walker WJ and Giddings AEB. Thrombolysis – a challenge for radiologists and surgeons. *Clin Radiol* 1990; **41**: 299–300
43. Berridge DC, Gregson RHS, Makin GS and Hopkinson BR. Tissue plasminogen activator in peripheral thrombolysis. *Br J Surg* 1990; **77**: 179–82
44. Eisenbud DE, Brener BJ, Shoenfeld R *et al*. Treatment of acute vascular occlusions with intra-arterial urokinase. *Am J Surg* 1990; **160**: 160–5
45. Durham JD, Geller SC, Abbott WM *et al*. Regional infusion of urokinase into occluded lower-extremity bypass grafts: long-term clinical results. *Radiology* 1989; **172**: 83–7
46. Berridge DC, Perkins AC and Frier M *et al*. Detection and characterization of arterial thromboses using a platelet-specific monoclonal antibody (P256 Fab'). *Br J Surg* 1991; **78**: 1130–3
47. Palmer RMJ, Ferrige AG and Moncada S. Nitric oxide release accounts for the biological activity of endothelium-derived relaxing factor. *Nature* 1987; **327**: 524–6
48. Wilson AR and Fuch JCA. Percutaneous transluminal angioplasty. The radiologist's contribution to the treatment of vascular disease. *Sur Clin North Am* 1984; **64**: 121–50
49. Hoylaerts M, Rijken DC, Lijnen HR, Collen D. Kinetics of the activation of plasminogen by human tissue plasminogen activator. *J Biol Chem* 1982; **257**: 2912–19
50. Eisert WG and Muller TH. Synergy in thrombolysis *in vivo* is species dependent (Abstr). *Circulation* 1987; **76**: IV–101
51. Collen D, Stump DC and Van de Werf F. Coronary thrombolysis in patients with acute myocardial infarction by intravenous infusion of synergistic thrombolytic agents. *Am Heart J* 1986; **112**: 1083–4
52. Collen D and Van de Werf F. Coronary arterial thrombolysis with low-dose synergistic combinations of recombinant tissue-type plasminogen activator (rt-PA) and recombinant single-chain urokinase-type plasminogen activator (rscu-PA) for acute myocardial infarction. *Am J Cardiol* 1987; **60**: 431–4
53. Topol EJ, Califf RM, George BS *et al*. Coronary arterial thrombolysis with combined infusion of recombinant tissue-type plasminogen activator and urokinase in acute myocardial infarction. *Circulation* 1988; **77**: 1100–7
54. Gardiner GA, Meyerovitz MF, Stokes KR, Clouse ME, Harrington DP and Bettmann MA. Complications of transluminal angioplasty. *Radiology* 1986; **159**: 201–8
55. Lonsdale RJ, Berridge DC, Earnshaw JJ *et al*. Recombinant tissue-type plasminogen activator is superior to streptokinase for local intra-arterial thrombolysis. *Br J Surg* 1992; **79**: 272–5

56. Harker LA. Role of platelets and thrombosis in mechanisms of acute occlusion and restenosis after angioplasty. *Am J Cardiol* 1987; **60**: 20B–28B

57. Block PC, Myler RK, Stertzer S and Fallon JT. Morphology after transluminal angioplasty in human beings. *New Engl J Med* 1981; **305**: 382–5

58. Cunningham DA, Kumar B, Siegel BA, Gilula LA, Totty WG and Welch MJ. Aspirin inhibition of platelet deposition at angioplasty sites: demonstration by platelet scintigraphy. *Radiology* 1984; **131**: 487–90

59. Lonsdale RJ, Perkins AC, Heptinstall S, Wenham PW, Makin GS and Hopkinson BR. Systemic platelet activation and local platelet deposition during angioplasty: a role for aspirin (Abstr). *Br J Surg* 1992; **79**: 359

60. Ameli FM, Stein M, Provan JL, St. Louis EL and Legrand L. Percutaneous transluminal angioplasty without anticoagulation. *Ann Vasc Surg* 1989; **3**: 244–7

61. Berridge DC, Earnshaw JJ, Westby JC, Makin GS and Hopkinson BR. Fibrinolytic profiles in local low-dose thrombolysis with streptokinase and recombinant tissue plasminogen activator. *Thromb Haemost* 1989; **61**: 275–8

62. Dotter CT and Judkins MP. Transluminal treatment of arteriosclerotic obstruction. Description of a new technic and a preliminary report of its application. *Circulation* 1964; **30**: 654–70

63. Clyne CAC, Archer TJ, Atuhaire LK, Chant ADS and Webster JHH. Random control trial of a short course of aspirin and dipyridamole (Persantin) for femorodistal grafts. *Br J Surg* 1987; **74**: 246–8

64. Green RM, Roedersheimer LR and DeWeese JA. Effects of aspirin and dipyridamole on expanded polytetrafluroethylene graft patency. *Surgery* 1982; **92**: 1016–26

65. McCollum C, Alexander C, Kenchington, G, Franks PJ and Greenhalgh R. Antiplatelet drugs in femoropopliteal vein bypasses: a multicenter trial. *J Vasc Surg* 1991; **13**: 150–62

66. Lowe GDO. Drugs in cerebral and peripheral arterial disease. *Br Med J* 1990; **300**: 524–8

67. Antiplatelet Trialists' Collaboration. Secondary prevention of vascular disease by prolonged antiplatelet treatment. *Br Med J* 1988; **296**: 320–31

68. Schumacher WA, Lee EC and Lucchesi BR. Augmentation of streptokinase-induced thrombolysis by heparin and prostacyclin. *J Cardiovasc Pharmacol* 1983; **7**: 739–46

69. Lammer J, Pilger E, Neumayer K and Schreyer H. Intraarterial fibrinolysis: long-term results. *Radiology* 1986; **161**: 159–63

70. Lonsdale RJ, Whitaker SC, Berridge DC *et al.* Peripheral arterial thrombolysis: intermediate-term results. *Br J Surg* 1993; **80**: 592–5

71. Browse DJ, Torrie EPH and Galland RB. Early results and 1 year follow up after intra-arterial thrombolysis. *Br J Surg* 1993; **80**: 194–7

Chapter 10

Intra-operative thrombolysis

J. D. Beard

Introduction

Percutaneous intra-arterial thrombolytic therapy is now well established for the treatment of acute leg ischaemia[1], and has also recently been used in acute arm ischaemia[2]. However, complete clot lysis may take many hours and so the technique is of little use when the limb is so severely ischaemic that immediate intervention is required. The treatment of choice in such cases remains thromboembolectomy using a balloon catheter[3,4]. Unfortunately this procedure fails to reperfuse the limb in a significant proportion of cases, resulting in amputation and/or death[5-7].

The technique of balloon catheter embolectomy has changed little since its introduction by Fogarty nearly 30 years ago[3]. Although it is a relatively simple method for removing thromboembolus it is not without problems. With the advancing age of the population, underlying atherosclerosis may complicate the situation even if the cause is embolic (Figure 10.1). Increasingly, acute thrombosis rather than embolism is the problem, especially in the leg[8].

Jivegard *et al.* retrospectively studied 236 acutely ischaemic legs treated by balloon catheter embolectomy alone[5]. They were able to establish with certainty a diagnosis of embolism in 92 and thrombosis in 30 cases. Failure to revascularize the leg was significantly more common in the group with thrombosis (50% vs 13%) and there was a correspondingly higher mortality rate (Figure 10.2).

Arterial damage by the embolectomy catheter is more likely if atherosclerosis is present, as stenoses prevent distal passage of the catheter. The catheter tip may cause an intimal dissection or complete perforation if passed vigorously[9] and endothelial denudation is likely if the balloon is over-inflated[10]. Even if acute thrombosis does not result, the endothelial injury may be a stimulus for late neointimal hyperplasia. Mechanical methods always fail to remove thromboembolus from small distal vessels or side branches. Experimental work in dogs has demonstrated the progression of thrombosis to arteries of the skin and muscle after 6 hours of arterial inflow occlusion[11]. Although irreversible tissue damage may not have occurred at this stage, it is inevitable if these arteries are not cleared.

Embolectomy is commonly performed 'blind' without radiological control despite several studies which have reported incomplete clearance of distal

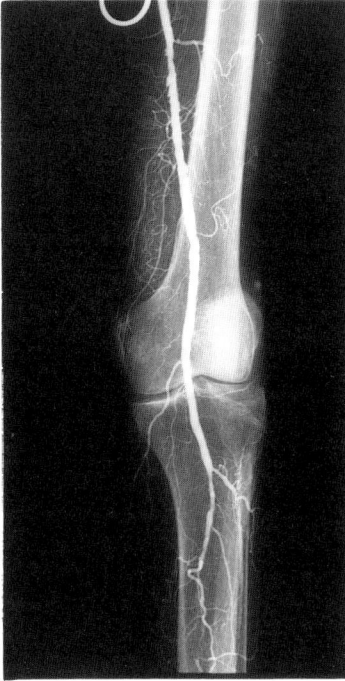

Figure 10.1 Completion angiogram following embolectomy for cardiac embolus. The superficial femoral artery and popliteal artery are patent but there is atheromatous disease distally

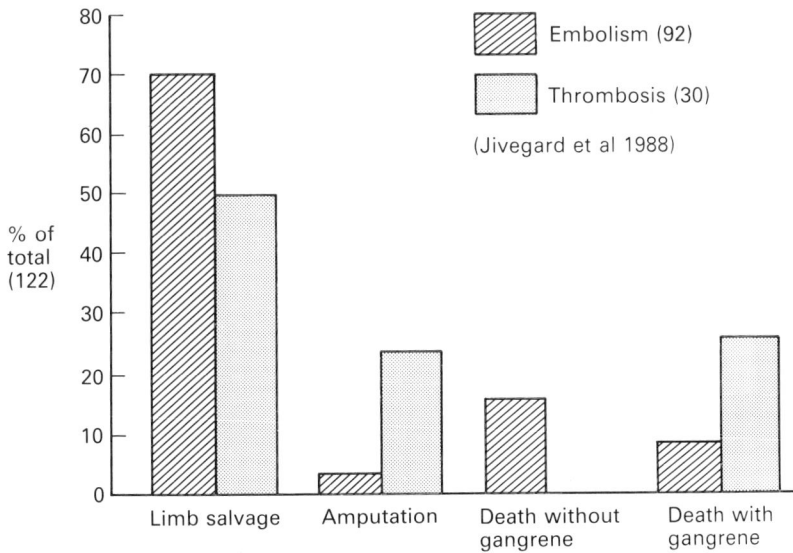

Figure 10.2 Comparison of the outcome after embolectomy of 122 acutely ischaemic legs due to embolism or thrombosis

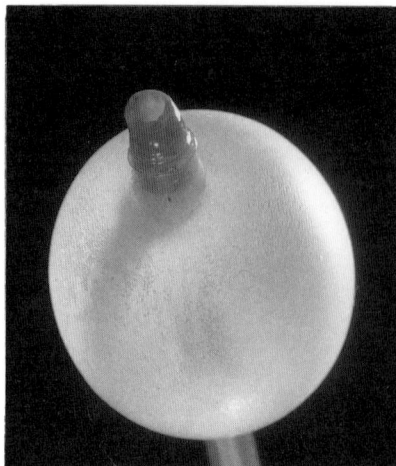

Figure 10.3 Combined irrigation/ embolectomy catheter with an end hole permitting passage over a guidewire and subsequent arteriography or lysis

thrombus in up to 30% of cases[12,13]. The results of embolectomy have been shown to be better when completion arteriography is performed[13,14]. When performing a femoral embolectomy, the catheter tends preferentially to enter the peroneal branch rather than the anterior or posterior tibial arteries[15] and a similar lack of direction can occur during brachial embolectomy[16]. The use of a combined irrigation/embolectomy catheter (Figure 10.3), passed over a guidewire, may permit selective catheterization of the distal branches and repeated arteriograms are also possible via the catheter[17].

A solution to the limitations of balloon catheter embolectomy is to combine it with intra-operative thrombolytic therapy. This permits rapid removal of the main bulk of the thrombus by a conventional balloon catheter, followed by lysis of any residue in the distal arteries and side branches. Intra-operative intra-arterial thrombolysis was first described by Cotton et al. in 1962[18]. Since then there have been several series reported from the USA[19–23], and one from the UK[24], using a variety of agents including streptokinase, urokinase and tissue plasminogen activator (t-PA).

Indications

Percutaneous intra-arterial thrombolysis is now the treatment of choice for many cases of acute limb ischaemia. There remain three indications for balloon catheter thromboembolectomy (plus intra-operative thrombolysis, where necessary):

1. Severe, acute limb ischaemia with a sensorimotor deficit.
2. Graft occlusion where catheter placement for percutaneous thrombolysis has not been possible or is contra-indicated.
3. Lack of availability or failure of percutaneous thrombolysis (Figure 10.4).

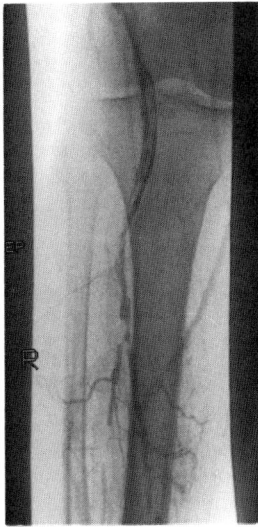

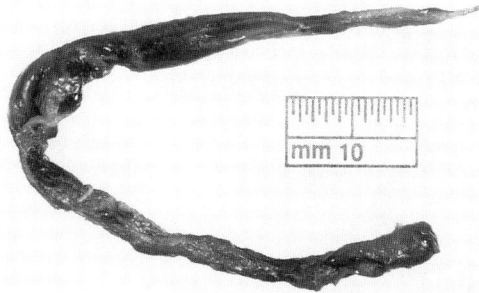

(b)

Figure 10.4 (a) Operative angiogram after percutaneous thrombolysis showing residual embolus. (b) Old organized embolus retrieved by balloon catheter embolectomy

(a)

If balloon catheter thromboembolectomy is performed, then it has been proposed that quality control to ensure complete clearance of clot is mandatory. Intra-operative arteriography is the best established method[12,13], but vascular endoscopy may be an acceptable alternative[25]. Intra-operative thrombolysis is indicated if residual thrombus is demonstrated. It is not always possible for the arteriogram to distinguish between residual thrombus and an atherosclerotic occlusion, and in equivocal cases a trial of thrombolysis is worth while as the alternative is a more distal arterial exploration or bypass graft.

Another possible indication for intra-operative rather than percutaneous thrombolysis is thrombosis of a popliteal aneurysm. Although percutaneous thrombolysis is now a well-established initial treatment[26], surgical repair or bypass of the aneurysm is required once the thrombus in the calf vessels has been lysed. Intra-operative thrombolysis of these run-off vessels combined with urgent surgical reconstruction has potential advantages in terms of speed and simplicity[27].

The acutely ischaemic limb with sensorimotor deficit is a surgical emergency and no time should be wasted in transferring the patient to the operating theatre. Pain should be treated with adequate narcotic analgesia and 5000 units of heparin given intravenously to reduce propagation of clot, as this has a beneficial effect on outcome[14].

Pre-operative arteriography is not usually necessary in severe ischaemia as it may delay treatment and in most cases the management is not altered[28]. There are a few exceptions to this statement. Most patients with an acutely ischaemic leg have a palpable femoral pulse even if the common femoral artery contains thrombus; the pulse may even be 'enhanced' due to lack of distal flow. If there is no femoral pulse an arteriogram should be considered if there is no risk factor for embolism. The cause may be an iliac thrombosis or dissection of the abdominal aorta, both of which are unlikely to be correctable by surgical exploration of the femoral artery. If both legs are acutely ischaemic with absent femoral pulses, then the cause is either a saddle embolus, aortic thrombosis or dissection. Arteriography should again be considered if there is no risk factor for embolism. The other indication for arteriography is suspected thrombosis/embolism of a popliteal aneurysm because percutaneous thrombolysis is a reasonable treatment option[26]. The best clue is palpation of the contralateral popliteal pulse as popliteal aneurysms are often bilateral. Ultrasound is also of value in confirming this diagnosis.

Method

Many techniques of intra-operative thrombolysis have been described using streptokinase, urokinase and t-PA[19-23]. The method described in detail here was that used by the author and his colleagues to treat 42 acutely ischaemic legs and two arms[24]. Our limited experience of intra-operative thrombolysis in the arm is due to the low incidence of upper limb acute ischaemia. Acute arm ischaemia is usually due to embolism[29] and the lack of underlying atherosclerosis normally ensures good clot clearance by balloon catheter alone. The method of intra-operative thrombolysis is described in conjunction with exploration of the femoral artery as this is the commonest site for surgical intervention in the acutely ischaemic limb but it is equally applicable elsewhere, including at popliteal and tibial artery level[30].

With the increasing age of the general population, co-existing atherosclerosis often complicates the situation even if the cause is purely embolic, especially in the leg. Complex secondary procedures may be necessary if embolectomy and intra-operative thrombolysis fails. It is therefore advisable that this operation be performed by an experienced vascular surgeon and there is evidence that better results are obtained by specialized units[31].

Exploration of the femoral artery

Both groins and the entire leg, except for the foot, should be prepared. This permits ease of access for arteriography and further surgery if required (Figure 10.5). The foot is placed in a clear plastic 'bowel bag' so that it can easily be inspected during the operation without the risk of desterilizing the operative field.

The common femoral artery and its bifurcation are exposed via a vertical groin incision. Care should be taken to preserve the lateral tributary of the long saphenous vein as it may be used later as a vein patch. The common femoral, superficial femoral and deep femoral arteries are controlled by silastic slings and the common femoral artery crossclamped if a strong pulse is present. Clamps should initially be avoided, if possible, because they may fragment thrombus which might otherwise be removed intact. A transverse arteriotomy is made in the common femoral artery just proximal to the bifurcation. An arteriotomy at the bifurcation should be avoided because an atheromatous plaque is often present here and the internal orifice of the deep femoral artery may be more proximal than it appears from the outside. It has been claimed that a longitudinal arteriotomy is advantageous if arterial

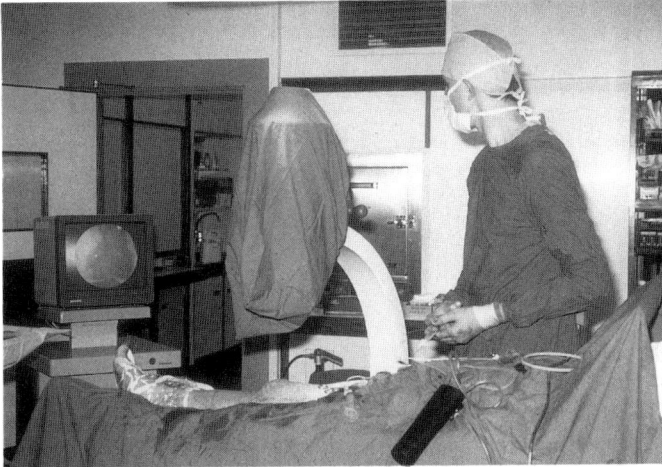

Figure 10.5 Perioperative arteriography using fluoroscopy. The entire leg is prepared for ease of access and the foot enclosed in a sterile bowel bag to allow inspection

reconstruction becomes necessary. However, a transverse incision is easier to close without narrowing the vessel and can be converted to a diamond-shaped incision if reconstruction is required.

On opening the artery, any thrombus at the bifurcation can be removed with gentle suction or fine artery forceps, and momentarily releasing the clamp often clears any proximal thrombus. If good pulsatile inflow is not present, then a 4 or 5F balloon catheter should be passed proximally up into the aorta, inflated and withdrawn. Pressure should be applied to the contra-lateral femoral artery during this procedure so that any thrombus dislodged over the aortic bifurcation passes into the internal iliac artery. If the catheter will not pass proximally and good inflow cannot be achieved, then the diagnosis is probably an iliac thrombosis or aortic dissection and a bypass will be required. An extra-anatomic bypass graft, e.g. femoro-femoral or axillo-bifemoral, avoids the hazard of direct aortic surgery[32]. A saddle embolus can usually be retrieved by bilateral balloon catheter embolectomy[33].

Once good inflow is secured, a 4F balloon catheter is passed as far distally as possible down both the deep and superficial femoral arteries. Force should not be used if resistance is met as dissection or perforation may result[9]. A 3F catheter should be tried instead. The balloon is inflated and the catheter withdrawn, adjusting balloon inflation and traction force to avoid damaging the artery[10]. The procedure is repeated until no further thromboembolic material can be retrieved.

Uncontrolled passage of a balloon catheter down the superficial femoral artery is limited because the surgeon has no control over its trajectory beyond the popliteal trifurcation. The catheter will tend to pass down the most direct branch which is often the peroneal artery[15]. Combined irrigation/embolectomy catheters permit selective passage over a guidewire under fluoroscopic control[17] and thrombus can also be removed this way (Figure 10.6).

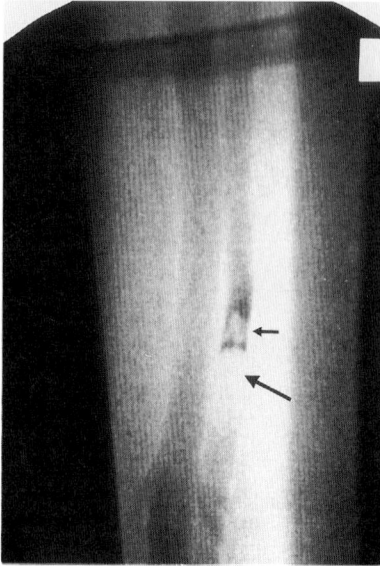

Figure 10.6 Retrieval of embolus (small arrow) from superficial femoral artery under fluoroscopic control using combined irrigation/embolectomy catheter (large arrow)

Intraoperative arteriography

A completion arteriogram should always be performed as significant thrombus may persist even if the catheter passes to the foot[12,13]. The presence of backbleeding is of no prognostic value as this merely indicates that the artery is patent down to the level of a collateral branch. Completion angiography has been shown to improve the results of embolectomy[14]. A film cassette wrapped in a sterile towel is placed under the leg from mid-thigh to mid-calf. Twenty millilitres of contrast medium is infused down the superficial femoral artery as quickly as possible via a Tibbs arterial cannula, or umbilical catheter, snugged into position using a silastic sling with the inflow clamped. The film is exposed as the injection ends (Figure 10.7). An end hole, combined embolectomy/irrigation catheter (Meadox, UK) can be used for embolectomy, arteriography and subsequent lysis. Arteriography or thrombolysis is simply performed using the irrigation channel after inflation of the balloon to prevent leakage.

The artery is then flushed with heparinized saline and if no thrombus is present on the arteriogram, the arteriotomy is closed. The arteriotomy should be closed with a running suture of 5/0 polypropylene from each end, with the needles passed from proximal to distal to avoid an intimal dissection. On removing the clamps, the foot should rapidly become pink with palpable pulses.

Fluoroscopy with image intensification is an excellent alternative to static angiography[34]. It avoids the problem of mistiming the contrast injection, permits thorough screening down to the foot and also saves development time. If fluoroscopy is to be used it is important to ensure that the patient is placed on an appropriate operating table with adequate clearance for the C-arm beneath the table legs. Fluoroscopy has the disadvantage of leaving

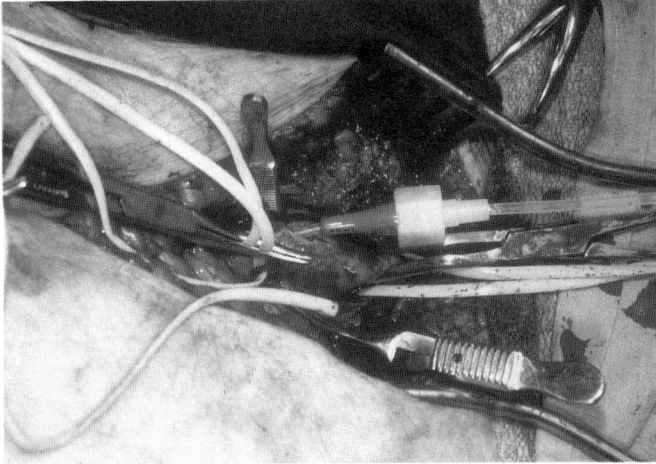

Figure 10.7 Operative arteriography and thrombolysis via an umbilical catheter fixed into the femoral artery with a silastic sling

no permanent record unless a hard-copy or video storage facility is available. Angioscopy may become an acceptable alternative in the future[25], but at present the instruments are delicate, expensive and offer no real advantage over arteriography. The large volume of irrigation fluid required during angioscopy may also cause problems in these patients who frequently suffer from cardiac insufficiency.

Intraoperative thrombolysis

If the arteriogram shows residual thrombus or complete occlusion of the distal vessels then 100 000 units of streptokinase in 100 ml heparinized saline is infused via the same cannula used for the arteriogram over a 30-minute period and the arteriogram repeated. This often demonstrates complete clot lysis (Figure 10.8). The streptokinase may be added to a 100 ml 'minibag' of normal saline, plus 1000 units of heparin, and infused under gravity, or via an infusion pump. A simpler method is to mix the streptokinase with 100 ml of heparinized saline from the scrub nurses' trolley and give it in 20 ml boluses at 5-minute intervals.

The reason for an infusion, rather than a single bolus, is that although the distal arteries are theoretically isolated, there will always be some collateral supply with leaching of the thrombolytic solution into the venous, and then systemic circulation. Unlike percutaneous thrombolysis, no attempt is made to embed the cannula or catheter into the thrombus. This is normally done to concentrate the thrombolytic agent within the thrombus which would otherwise be rapidly washed away by flowing blood. Cohen et al.[19] used the embedding technique intra-operatively to no obvious advantage. In this static situation it is probably unnecessary, especially as the thrombus has already been partially fragmented by the balloon catheter, though it is wise to leave the catheter tip as close to the clot as possible.

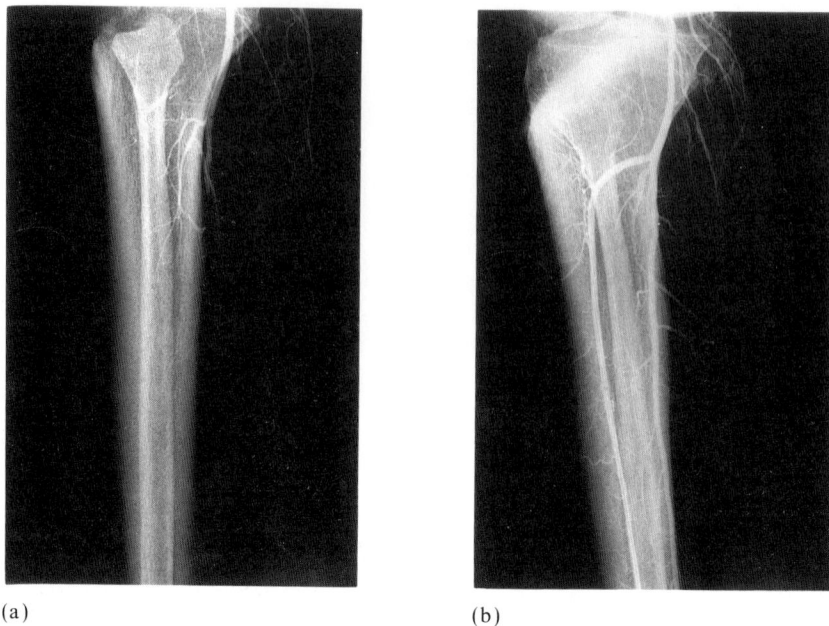

(a)   (b)

Figure 10.8 (a) Residual occlusion of the popliteal artery after embolectomy despite repeated passage of the catheter to the ankle. (b) Complete lysis following 100 000 units streptokinase

If the subsequent arteriogram shows incomplete lysis, then it is worth passing the balloon catheter again as the thrombus may have become less adherent[20] (Figure 10.9). A second infusion of 100 000 units of streptokinase may be given intra-operatively though larger doses risk significant side effects[24]. Alternatively, a low-dose streptokinase infusion via a catheter inserted into a side branch may be continued post-operatively[30,34]. Rapid lysis has been reported using two boluses of 5 mg t-PA at 10-minute intervals[35], but the possible advantage may be outweighed by the high cost of t-PA. Use of t-PA is certainly indicated if the patient has received streptokinase in the previous year – more due to the presence of neutralizing anti-streptococcal antibodies than the risk of anaphylaxis[36]. Presumably other thrombolytic agents such as urokinase would be equally effective though the optimal dose is not known. Fibrin specificity is unlikely to be an advantage in this situation.

Comerota et al.[23] have recently described an isolated limb perfusion technique which permits the use of high doses of thrombolytic agents during surgery without the risk of systemic effects. After draining the leg of venous blood by elevation and a compression bandage, a thigh tourniquet is inflated to 350 mmHg. The distal popliteal vein is cannulated with a catheter via a transverse venotomy and catheters also passed down the anterior and posterior tibial arteries via the popliteal artery. After infusion of 500 000 units of urokinase down each tibial artery, the limb is flushed with heparinized saline until the venous effluent runs clear. The venotomy is closed primarily and the arteriotomy closed with a vein patch.

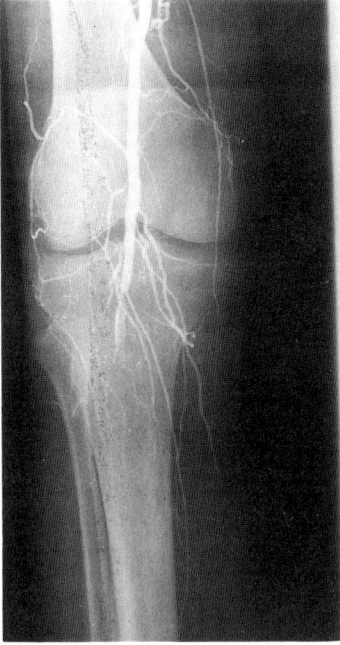

(a)

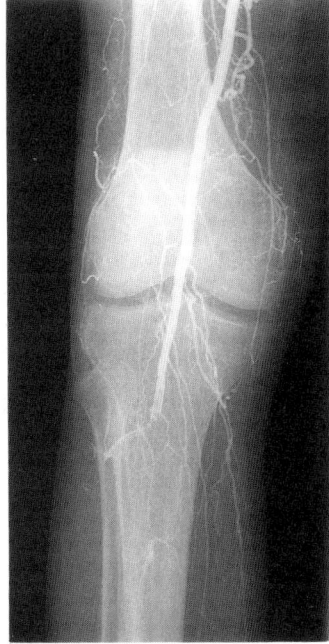

(b)

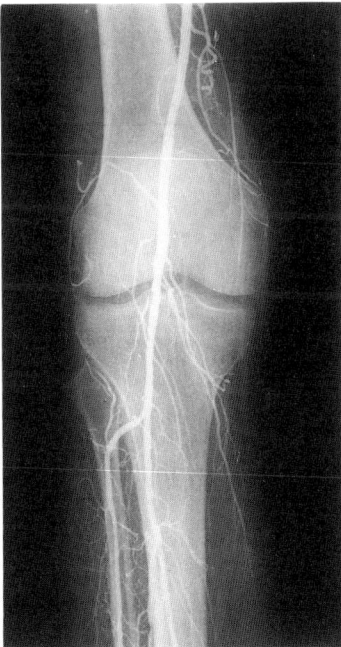

(c)

Figure 10.9 (a) Popliteal artery occlusion after embolectomy. (b) Following streptokinase infusion there is some improvement with loosening of thrombus. (c) Complete clearance after repeat embolectomy

Further management

There is little reason why fresh thromboembolic material should not be lysed rapidly by any thrombolytic agent. Incomplete or no lysis is likely to signify the presence of old, organized thrombus or atheroma requiring mechanical removal or bypass (Figure 10.10).

If an underlying stenosis of the superficial femoral artery is revealed after thrombolysis, then intra-operative angioplasty may be tried if the surgeon has experience with this technique (Figure 10.11). Persistent occlusion will necessitate exploration of the popliteal artery and trifurcation via a medial below-knee incision. A longitudinal arteriotomy is used at this site and proximal embolectomy using a 4 or 3F balloon catheter may be successful in clearing thrombus from the distal superficial femoral artery. A 3 or 2F balloon catheter can be passed down the individual calf arteries but frequently the trifurcation is found to be severely diseased. Intra-operative thrombolysis can again be performed down the individual tibial arteries, in divided doses, using the popliteal arteriotomy. This is particularly useful when dealing with an acutely thrombosed popliteal aneurysm where the run off is frequently compromised by thromboembolic material[27]. The arteriotomy requires a vein patch repair to prevent narrowing.

If the underlying problem is persistent thrombotic occlusion of the distal superficial femoral or popliteal artery, due to atheroma or aneurysm, then a bypass graft will be required[32]. Poor calf vessel run off is a more difficult problem. Whilst it is probably unnecessary, although good practice, to aim for clearance of all three vessels, the absence of a single vessel in continuity with the plantar arch carries a poor prognosis. Although a trial of reperfusion is perfectly acceptable, the surgeon should be prepared to explore the tibial arteries at ankle level if required. An aggressive policy of ankle level embolectomy, thrombolysis and, when required, femoro-distal bypass grafting has been reported to increase limb salvage rates[30].

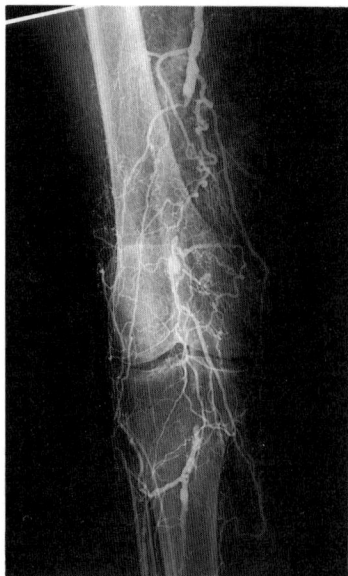

Figure 10.10 Operative angiogram after failed attempt to pass a balloon catheter down the superficial femoral artery. Intra-operative thrombolysis had no effect upon this lesion which turned out to be an atherosclerotic occlusion. Surgical bypass was required

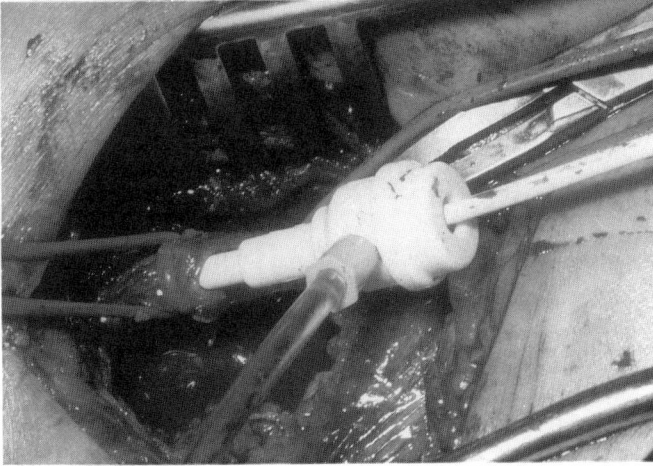

Figure 10.11 Operative angioplasty using a sheath inserted into the femoral arteriotomy. The sheath has a valve that permits removal and exchange of catheters without blood loss and also reduces trauma to the vessel wall

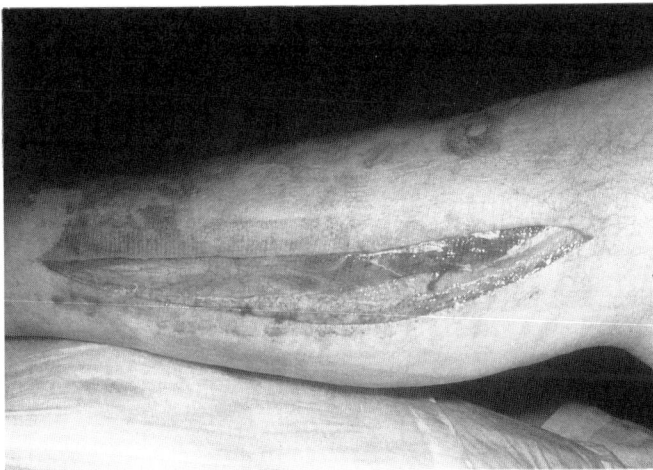

Figure 10.12 Full-length fasciotomy of the lower leg following femoral embolectomy and operative thrombolysis. The severity of the ischaemia is evidenced by the pale, bulging muscle and skin staining

Revascularization of ischaemic muscle can result in considerable swelling within the fascial compartments of the leg, especially if ischaemia has been prolonged. This compartment syndrome will lead to further ischaemic damage if not relieved[37]. Failed percutaneous thrombolysis, in particular, carries a significant risk of this. A fasciotomy from knee to ankle should be performed if there is any tension or swelling of the calf muscles. Although decompression of all three compartments, by excision of the fibula, has been advocated following trauma, an antero-lateral and postero-medial fasciotomy is more practical in thromboembolic disease (Figure 10.12). If the circulation cannot adequately be restored despite thrombolysis and/or distal reconstruction, immediate amputation should be considered as it may be life-saving[28], though there are problems if informed consent has not been obtained pre-operatively.

Results

During the past 5 years we have used intra-operative thrombolysis in 42 acutely ischaemic legs after intra-operative arteriography demonstrated residual thrombus or persistent occlusion following balloon catheter embolectomy. There were 41 patients (23 men and 18 women) aged 42–86 years (median 76), which reflects the advanced age and frailty of many of these patients. The indication for operation was severe ischaemia with sensorimotor deficit in 32, failed percutaneous thrombolysis in six, and four cases where an occluded prosthetic bypass graft was not accessible to percutaneous thrombolysis.

The cause of the ischaemia was probably a spontaneous embolus in 13 cases (11 of cardiac origin, one aortic plaque and one aortic aneurysm); thrombosis of an atherosclerotic stenosis in 12; a thrombosed popliteal aneurysm in five; graft occlusion in six (one femoro-femoral, one ilio-femoral and four femoro-popliteal PTFE grafts), and iatrogenic embolism in six cases (five following percutaneous angioplasty and one after aortic surgery). The differentiation between spontaneous embolism and thrombosis was made on the basis of pre-operative risk factors (ECG evidence of arrhythmia or myocardial infarction, a past history of claudication and the presence of contra-lateral pulses); arteriographic and operative findings; plus histology and autopsy results, where applicable.

The primary operative procedures, before intra-operative thrombolysis, are summarized in Figure 10.13(a). A femoral embolectomy was performed in just under half of the cases (48%); a popliteal embolectomy in 28%; combined femoral and popliteal approaches in 9.5%; graft thrombectomy in 12%; and combined graft and femoral exploration in one case. Following femoral embolectomy, the usual site of residual thrombus or occlusion on the post-embolectomy arteriogram was the popliteal artery or trifurcation (Figure 10.8). In most cases this level corresponded to the point beyond which the catheter could not be passed. However, on 11 occasions proximal thrombus or occlusion was found even though the catheter had been successfully passed to the ankle.

The post-streptokinase arteriogram demonstrated complete lysis in 21 legs (50%), (Figures 10.14 and 10.15); partial lysis in a further 13 (31%); and no change in eight (19%). Of the eight that showed no change, the occlusion was found to be due to pre-existing atherosclerosis (Figure 10.10), rather than thrombus in five cases where popliteal exploration or post-mortem examination was undertaken. The other three were unproven, but there was not a single case of proven thrombus that was not at least partially lysed by streptokinase. Additional procedures largely depended upon the degree of lysis (Figure 10.13(b)). Nothing further was done in 20 cases (48%) and exploration was thereby avoided. In cases of incomplete lysis, repeat embolectomy succeeded in clearing remaining thrombus from the popliteal

PRIMARY PROCEDURE (42)

(a)

ADDITIONAL PROCEDURE (22/42)

(b)

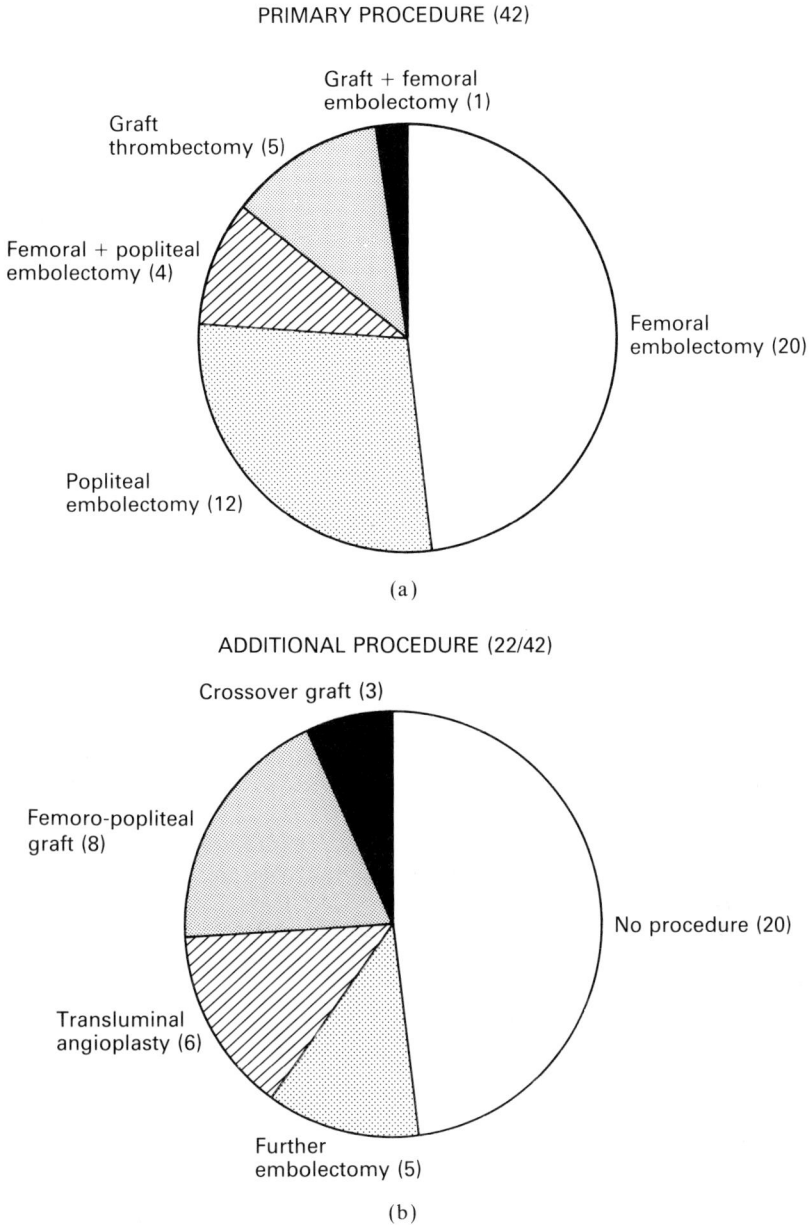

Figure 10.13 Intra-operative thrombolysis after failed embolectomy in 42 cases. (a) Primary operative procedure before arteriography. (b) Additional operative procedures after intra-operative streptokinase

artery on five occasions, due to loosening (Figure 10.9), but further doses of streptokinase were invariably ineffective. Transluminal balloon angioplasty of an underlying stenosis was performed in six cases (14%), and bypass grafts were required in 11 (26%). Of these, three were femoro-femoral cross-over

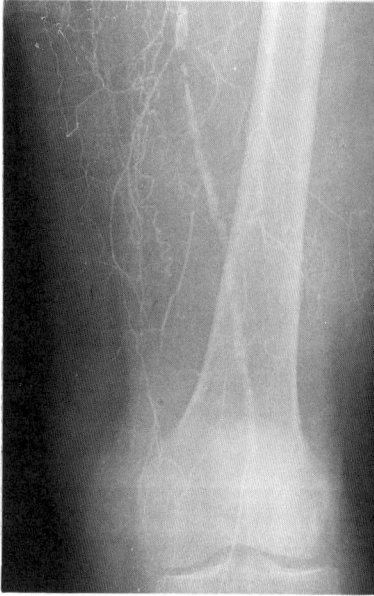

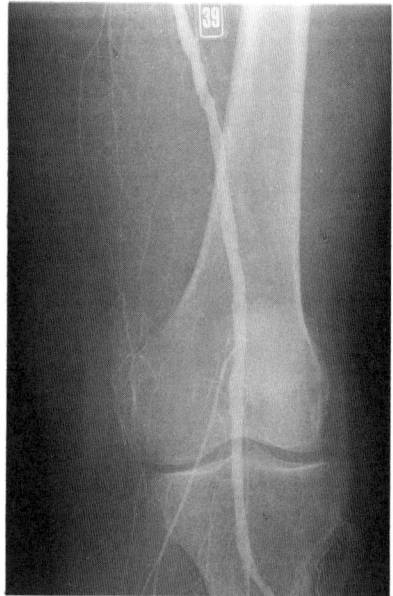

(a)   (b)

Figure 10.14 (a) Operative angiogram showing residual adherent thrombus in the superficial femoral artery after embolectomy. (b) Complete lysis following intra-operative streptokinase

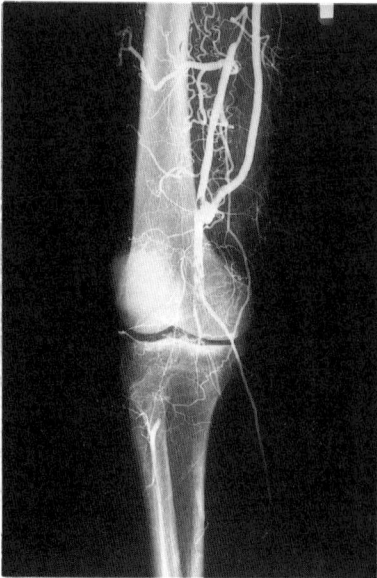

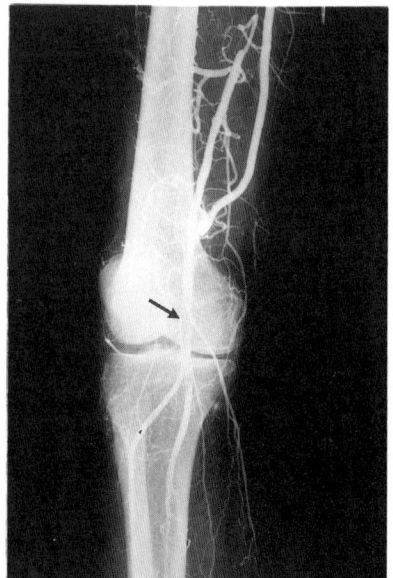

(a)   (b)

Figure 10.15 (a) Operative angiogram after balloon catheter thrombectomy of an above-knee PTFE graft. Good graft clearance but residual popliteal artery occlusion. (b) Repeat arteriogram after intra-operative streptokinase showing complete lysis with an underlying stenosis at the level of the knee joint which required angioplasty (arrow)

grafts because of poor inflow and eight were femoro distal grafts to bypass atherosclerotic occlusions or popliteal aneurysm. Anterior and posterior fasciotomy was performed in nine legs (21%).

The results, subdivided according to the cause of ischaemia, are summarized in Figure 10.16. The outcome for spontaneous embolism or thrombosis of a popliteal aneurysm was excellent, with complete or partial lysis in all 18 cases, restoration of pedal pulses in 15 (83%), and limb salvage in all cases. The results for atherosclerotic thrombosis or graft occlusion were encouraging with complete or partial lysis in 14 (78%), limb salvage in 12 (67%), and were better if not compounded by poor calf vessel run off. Iatrogenic emboli, which are often composed of atherosclerotic rather than thrombotic material, fared badly. There was no case of complete lysis and a viable leg was only achieved in three cases (50%). Streptokinase was sometimes able to lyse the propagated thrombus in the larger arteries but if cholesterol microembolism had occurred (Figure 10.17), tissue perfusion did not improve[38]. Embolectomy was repeated in six legs that re-thrombosed postoperatively due to poor run off or atheromatous emboli but none was salvaged. A characteristic radiological sign in these non-viable limbs is extravasation of contrast or arteriovenous shunting giving a tufted appearance (Figure 10.18).

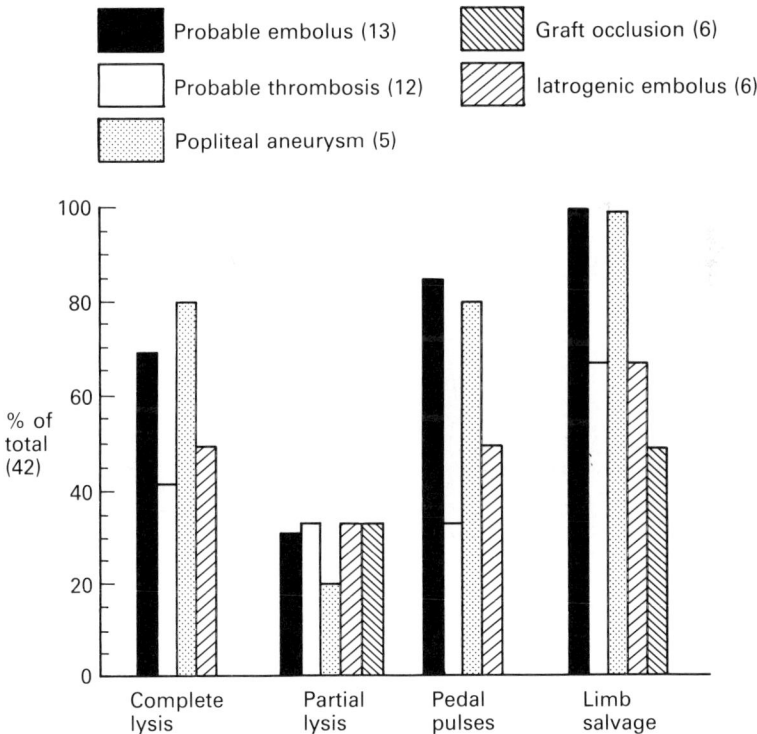

Figure 10.16 Results of intra-operative thrombolysis in 42 legs subdivided according to the cause of ischaemia

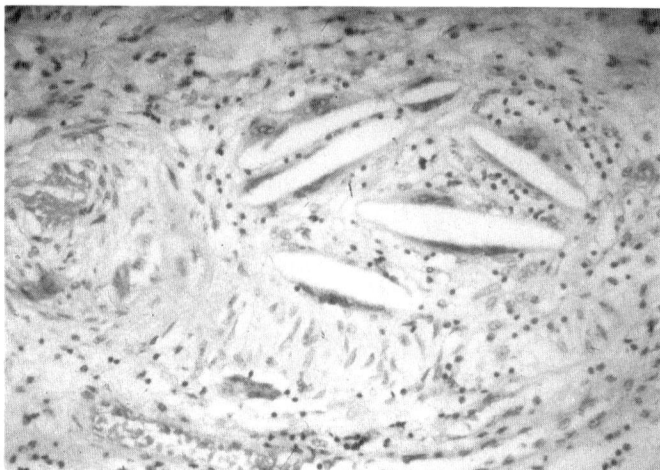

Figure 10.17 Cholesterol emboli lodged in a small artery resulting in acute thrombosis and an intense granulomatous reaction

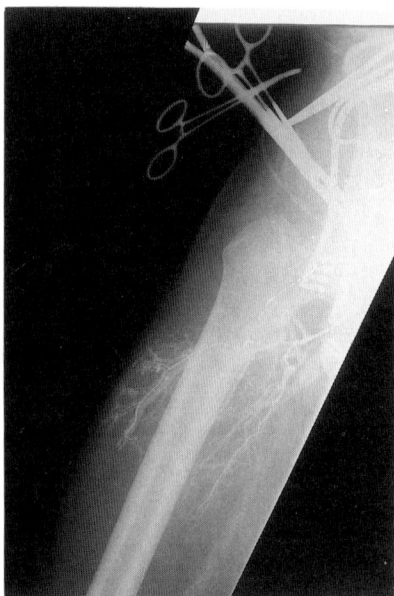

Figure 10.18 Operative angiogram in irreversible ischaemia due to cholesterol embolization. Characteristic tufting due to arteriovenous shunting

Post-operatively, at least one pedal pulse was restored in 23 legs (55%) and limb salvage achieved in 34 (81%) at the time of discharge or death. Doppler ankle pressures were not performed in all cases but are not particularly useful in acute limb ischaemia because frequently no signal can be detected prior to treatment. There was a significant correlation between successful lysis and restoration of pedal pulses (Fisher Exact Test: $P = 0.0031$) and a similar correlation with leg viability (Fisher Exact Test: $P = 0.0135$).

All patients were anti-coagulated with heparin in the post-operative period and converted to warfarin if in atrial fibrillation[39]. There were eight wound haematomas of which two required drainage but it is difficult to say whether these were associated with the administration of intra-operative streptokinase or related to the heparin. Complete coagulation profiles were not obtained in all patients, but two of the eight patients with haematomas had a low plasma fibrinogen suggesting systemic fibrinolysis. It should be noted that there were no bleeding problems in eight of the nine legs with fasciotomies. Two above-knee and two below-knee amputations were required, but none was in the successful lysis group. There were seven deaths, five of which were cardiac in origin (three myocardial infarction, two heart failure), which reflects the high incidence of ischaemic heart disease in these patients[40]. The other two were due to bronchopneumonia following an above-knee amputation and a stroke 10 days post-operatively.

Others have reported results of intra-operative thrombolytic therapy[19–23] (Table 10.1). Cohen et al.[19], in one of the earliest series, used 25–250 00 units of streptokinase in 11 legs after passing a catheter down into the clot, with successful lysis in 84%. In 1988, Norem et al.[20] reported the use of boluses of streptokinase or urokinase in 26 legs to lyse residual thrombus following femoral embolectomy. All had angiographic evidence of clot lysis, although this was combined with repeat embolectomy, resulting in a limb salvage of 85%.

Quinones-Baldrich et al.[21] reported the use of an intra-operative infusion of streptokinase or urokinase in 23 legs with lysis in 76% of those that had a repeat arteriogram (17), and limb salvage in 87%. Similar results have been reported by Parent et al.[22] but although both appeared equally effective, streptokinase was associated with more bleeding problems than urokinase. Comerota et al.[23] reported a series of 38 limbs including four arms and two cases of isolated limb perfusion. Their results are difficult to interpret but suggest a 47% lysis and 60% limb salvage rate. More recently, improved results using 10 mg t-PA have been suggested in a small series by Chester et al.[35], with 100% lysis in six legs. Wyffels et al.[30] have reported remarkable results for aggressive tibial artery embolectomy and thrombolysis at ankle level, with 100% lysis and limb salvage rates in 12 legs, although lysis was usually only achieved after additional post-operative thrombolytic infusions.

Table 10.1 Previously reported experience with intra-operative thrombolysis with streptokinase (SK), urokinase (UK) and t-PA, including the present series for comparison

Reference	Number	Agent	Lysis (%)	Salvage (%)
Cohen, 1986[19]	13	SK	84	64
Quinones, 1988[21]	23	SK/UK	76	87
Norem, 1988[20]	26	SK/UK	100	85
Parent, 1989[22]	17	SK/UK	88	—
Comerota, 1989[23]	38	SK/UK	47	60
Wyffels, 1992[30]	12	UK	17	100
Chester, 1992[35]	6	t-PA	100	—
Present series[24]	42	SK	81	81

Summary

The management of acute lower limb ischaemia is complex and should be performed by vascular surgeons in co-operation with vascular radiologists if good results are to be obtained. Although percutaneous thrombolytic therapy is a great advance, surgery is still required if it fails, or when there is severe ischaemia with sensorimotor deficit. This situation may change with the advent of percutaneous catheter aspiration of thrombus and quicker lysis times using pulsed spray techniques.

Femoral embolectomy remains an excellent way of removing large quantities of clot rapidly but completion arteriography is essential. Intra-operative thrombolysis is a safe and effective method of lysing any residual thrombus. Although this technique may avoid more distal arterial explora-tion, the surgeon must be prepared to proceed to popliteal exploration and distal reconstruction if necessary. Unfortunately, death due to concomitant cardiac disease will still occur but fewer patients should die as a result of inadequate revascularization.

References

1. Earnshaw JJ. Thrombolytic therapy in the management of acute limb ischaemia. *Br J Surg* 1991; **73**: 261–9
2. Willis DM, Venbrux AC, Benati JF, Mitchell SE, Lynch-Nyhan, A, Cassiday FP and Osterman FA. Fibrinolytic therapy for upper extremity arterial occlusions. *Radiology* 1990; **175**: 393–9
3. Fogarty TJ, Daily PO, Shumway NE and Krippachne W. Experience with balloon catheter technique for arterial embolectomy. *Am J Surg* 1971; **122**: 231–7
4. Blaisdell FW, Steele M and Allen RE. Management of acute lower extremity arterial ischaemia due to embolism and thrombosis. *Surgery* 1978; **84**: 822–34
5. Jivegard L, Holm J and Schersten T. The outcome of arterial embolism. *Acta Chir Scand* 1986; **152**: 251–6
6. Dregelid EB, Stangeland LB, Eide GE and Trippestaed A. Patient survival and limb prognosis after arterial embolectomy. *Eur J Vasc Surg* 1987; **1**: 263–71
7. Murie JA and Mathieson M. Arterial embolectomy in the leg: results in a referral hospital. *J Cardiovasc Surg* 1987; **28**: 184–8
8. Hight, DW, Tilney NI and Couch NP. Changing clinical trends in patients with peripheral arterial emboli. *Surgery* 1976; **79**: 172–6
9. Foster JH, Carter JW, Graham CP and Edwards WH. Arterial injuries secondary to the use of the Fogarty catheter. *Ann Surg* 1970; **171**: 971–8
10. Byrnes G and MacGowan WA. The injury potential of the Fogarty balloon catheter. *J Cardiovasc Surg* 1975; **175**: 590–3
11. Dunnant JH and Edwards WS. Small vessel occlusion in the extremity after various periods of arterial obstruction: an experimental study. *Surgery* 1973; **75**: 240–5
12. Mavor GE, Walker MG and Dhall DP. Routine operative arteriography in arterial embolectomy. *Br J Surg* 1972; **59**: 482–4
13. Bosma HW and Jorning PJG. Intraoperative arteriography in arterial embolectomy. *Eur J Vasc Surg* 1990; **4**: 469–72
14. Englund R and Magee HR. Peripheral arterial embolism: 1961–1985. *Aust NZ J Surg* 1987; **57**: 27–31
15. Short D, Vaughn GD and Jachimczyk J *et al*. The anatomic basis for the occasional failure of transfemoral balloon catheter thromboembolectomy. *Ann Surg* 1979; **190**: 555–6
16. Beckingham IJ, Roberts SNG, Berridge DC, Makin GS Hopkinson BR. A simple technique for thromboembolectomy of the upper limb. *Eur J Vasc Surg* 1990; **4**: 173–7

17. Robiczek F. Dye-enhanced fluoroscopy – directed catheter embolectomy. *Surgery* 1984; **95**: 622–4
18. Cotton LT, Flute PT and Tsapogas MJC. Popliteal artery thrombosis treated with streptokinase. *Lancet* 1962; **ii**: 1081–3
19. Cohen H, Kaplan M and Bernhard VM. Intraoperative streptokinase. An adjunct to mechanical thrombectomy in the management of acute ischaemia. *Arch Surg* 1986; **121**: 708–15
20. Norem RF, Short DH and Kerstein MD. Role of intraoperative fibrinolytic therapy in acute arterial occlusion. *Surg Gynecol Obstet* 1988; **167**: 87–91
21. Quinones-Baldrich WJ, Baker D, Busuttil RW and Machleder HI. Intraoperative infusion of lytic drugs for thrombotic complications of revascularization. *J Vasc Surg* 1989; **10**: 408–17
22. Parent FN, Bernhard VM, Pabst TS, McIntyre KE, Hunter GC and Malone JM. Fibrinolytic treatment of residual thrombus after catheter embolectomy for severe lower limb ischaemia. *J Vasc Surg* 1989; **9**: 153–60
23. Comerota AJ, White JV and Grosh JD. Intra-operative intra-arterial thrombolytic therapy for salvage of limbs in patients with distal arterial thrombosis. *Surg Gynecol Obstet* 1989; **169**: 283–9
24. Beard JD, Nyamekye I, Earnshaw JJ, Scott DJ and Thompson JF. Intraoperative streptokinase: a useful adjunct to balloon catheter embolectomy. *Br J Surg* 1993; **80**: 21–4
25. Grundfest WS, Litvack F, Glick D, Segalowitz J, Treiman R, Cohen L, Foran R, Levin P, Cossman D, Carroll R, Spiegelman A and Forrester JS. Intraoperative decisions based on angioscopy in peripheral vascular surgery. *Circulation* 1988; **78**: 114–17
26. Bowyer RC, Cawthorne SJ, Walker WJ and Giddings AFB. Conservative management of asymptomatic popliteal aneurysms. *Br J Surg* 1990; **71**: 1132–5
27. Thompson JF, Beard JD, Scott DJA and Earnshaw JJ. Intraoperative thrombolysis in the management of thrombosed popliteal aneurysm. *Br J Surg* 1993; **80**: 858–9
28. Scott DJ, Davies AH and Horrocks M. Risk factors in selected patients undergoing femoral embolectomy. *Ann R Coll Surg Engl* 1989; **71**: 229–32
29. Abbott WM, Mahoney RD, McCabe CC, Lee CE and Wirthin LS. Arterial embolism: a 44 year perspective. *Am J Surg* 1982; **143**: 460–4
30. Wyffels PL, Debord JR, Marshall JS, Thors G and Marshall WH. Increased limb salvage with intraoperative and postoperative ankle level urokinase infusion in acute lower limb ischaemia. *J Vasc Surg* 1992; **15**: 771–9
31. Clason AE, Stonebridge PA, Duncan AJ, Nolan B, Jenkins AMcL and Ruckley CV. Acute ischaemia of the lower limb: the effect of centralizing vascular surgical services on morbidity and mortality. *Br J Surg* 1989; **76**: 592–3
32. Hickey NC, Crowson MC and Simms MH. Emergency arterial reconstruction for acute ischaemia. *Br J Surg* 1990; **77**: 680–1
33. Ross SA, Hood JM and Barros D'Sa. Immediate heparinisation and surgery in the management of saddle embolism. *Eur J Vasc Surg* 1990; **4**: 191–4
34. Early GL and Hannah H. A technique for post embolectomy streptokinase infusion. *Arch Surg* 1985; **120**: 1395–7
35. Chester JF, Dormandy JA and Taylor RS. Peroperative tissue plasminogen activator thrombolysis as an adjunct to surgery. *Br J Surg* 1992; **79**: 366
36. Jalihal S and Morris GK. Antistreptokinase titres after intravenous streptokinase. *Lancet* 1990; **335**: 184–5
37. Ernst CB. Fasciotomy in perspective. *J Vasc Surg* 1990; **9**: 829–30
38. Gaines PA, Kennedy A, Moorhead P, Cumberland DC, Welsh CL and Rutley MS. Cholesterol embolisation: a lethal complication of vascular catheterisation. *Lancet* 1988; **ii**: 169–70
39. Hammarsten J, Holm and Shersten T. Positive and negative effects of anticoagulant treatment during and after arterial embolectomy. *J Cardiovasc Surg* 1978; **19**: 373–9
40. Clason AE, Stonebridge PA, Duncan AJ, Nolan B, Jenkins AM and Ruckley CV. Morbidity and mortality in acute lower limb ischaemia: a 5-year review. *Eur J Vasc Surg* 1975; **175**: 590–3

Chapter 11

Peripheral thrombolysis: state of the art

J. J. Earnshaw

The previous chapters have been written by authors very familiar with thrombolytic techniques who are responsible for the organization of a service in their own hospitals. Many different techniques and regimens have been presented which document the depth of knowledge and experience held by these clinicians. How can the optimal methods be decided when there is such variation over so many parts of the technique and so many different viewpoints are held. For example, in Guildford low-dose thrombolysis is only performed in the Intensive Care Unit, whereas at The Royal Free Hospital a vascular ward is used. At St. George's, accelerated lysis was developed so that the entire procedure could be carried out during a single visit to X-ray, thus avoiding this problem[1]. Some clinicians such as those at Guildford have opted for consistency of technique[2]. Others have found new methods and catheter technology irresistible and have changed their methods frequently from one to another. The result is a large number of small clinical trials published from individual units of uncontrolled or non-randomized investigations (Figure 11.1). Though some conclusions can be drawn from this information, it will take larger and more carefully co-ordinated studies before the art of peripheral thrombolysis can become a science.

Information from non-randomized trials

There is no doubt that the pattern of acute leg ischaemia has changed and become more technically challenging. The population at risk is elderly, often with associated atherosclerosis, and the situation of a pure embolism in otherwise normal vessels is a rarity. Treatment by the non-specialist is no longer acceptable[3] and for the best results experienced vascular surgeons and radiologists are required to work as a team[4]. Training of interventional vascular radiologists must include experience with thrombolytic techniques. It would also be ideal for trainee vascular surgeons to have some experience of endovascular techniques in an X-ray department and future training programmes should include this.

There is no doubt that thrombolytic therapy is effective in selected cases of acute leg ischaemia. Successive surveys over the past few years document

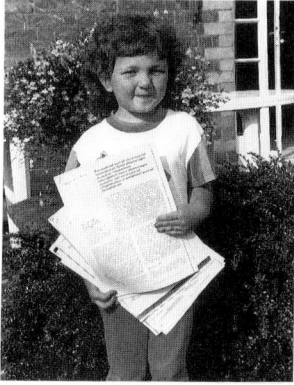
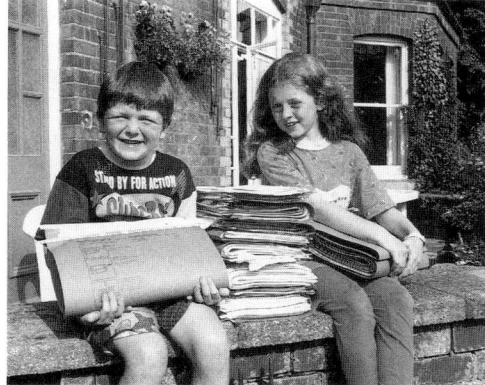

(a)   (b)

Figure 11.1 (a) Paucity of randomized trials in peripheral thrombosis. (b) Huge published literature on open clinical studies in peripheral thrombolysis

increasing experience with, and use of thrombolysis[5,6]. Most clinicians who report their results present a favourable overall message and it is remarkable how similar are the results from different institutions. There is a learning curve to using peripheral thrombolysis for acute leg ischaemia and results improve partly with experience and partly with case selection[7]. The duration of thrombolysis often reduces as a result of this experience which may account for improved results in sequential series from the same institution using different techniques. It is interesting that units with the greatest experience report a second trough or deterioration in results after an initial improvement. This is thought to be due to a relaxed case selection increasing the number of high-risk cases undertaken.

There is enormous variation in the reports on thrombolysis in the literature. There is still a problem with the definition of acute leg ischaemia and objective assessment of results and complications. Working parties of vascular surgeons and radiologists have addressed this problem in chronic critical leg ischaemia but much work needs to be undertaken in acute leg ischaemia before standardized reporting can be achieved. It is also clear from published reports that there are identifiable groups of patients in whom the chance of successful thrombolysis is increased.

Age

Increasing age is a significant determinant in the outcome from thrombolysis. To some extent this is a pure chronological problem though it is also due to the association of severe cardio-respiratory disease and general medical debility. In some elderly patients acute leg ischaemia is a pre-terminal event and in these cases treatment with either thrombolysis or surgery is unhelpful. It is a mistake to treat these patients actively but to recognize that conservative management is the kindest and most appropriate care.

Table 11.1 Post-mortem results in acute leg ischaemia ($n = 30$)

Clinical source	Post-mortem source
Potential embolic sources in patients thought to have died following embolism ($n = 8$)	
Atrial fibrillation (7)	Aortic atheroma (3)
Bilateral emboli (1)	Thoracic aneurysm (2)
	Mitral valve disease (1)
	None (2)
Potential embolic sources in patients thought to have died following thrombosis ($n = 22$)	
Atrial fibrillation (3)	Myocardial infarction (9)
Myocardial infarction (3)	(With mural thrombus – 3)
Cardiac arrhythmia (2)	Aortic atheroma (4)
None (14)	Multiple emboli (2)
	None (7)

Cause of occlusion

Some series report improved results of peripheral thrombolysis in patients with arterial emboli. Others feel that treatment of patients with emboli is contra-indicated, partly because there is the risk of further embolization from the primary source but also because treatment of old organized embolus which may not lyse is less logical than acute thrombus. Much of an arterial occlusion due to embolism is secondary thrombus which is, however, easy to lyse. It is doubtful whether it is possible to tell the difference between thrombus and embolus clinically.

A post-mortem study was undertaken in Nottingham to determine whether the pre-operative diagnosis of thrombus or embolus could be confirmed. In a series of 157 patients with acute leg ischaemia 33 died and 30 had post-mortems. Taking into account all information gathered from history, angiography and surgical exploration, patients were categorized into two diagnostic groups – embolus ($n = 8$) or thrombus ($n = 22$). At post-mortem, sources of emboli were sought in each group (Table 11.1). A possible source of embolus was found in 15 of the 22 patients thought to have thromboses and no source was identified in two of the eight patients thought to have had emboli. The conclusion was that it is not possible clinically to determine whether thrombus or embolus is the cause of acute leg ischaemia. What is termed embolus, i.e. a sudden onset of ischaemia in patients with normal vessels, may simply be a condition which responds well to surgical embolectomy whether the aetiology is thrombosis or embolism. In other words, thromboembolectomy works best in (relatively) normal arteries. Thus distinction between the two categories may be irrelevant and it is more logical to base management on the severity of the ischaemia rather than the cause.

Severity of ischaemia/length of occlusion/distal run off

Patients with severe ischaemia often have long arterial occlusions with poor run off. All these features are interlinked and carry a poor prognosis. The

Table 11.2 Definitions of acute leg ischaemia

A. Bell *et al.*[8] Working Party of the International Vascular Symposium

—Acute arrest of the circulation in a limb which was previously normal
—Persistent objective evidence of motor and sensory loss
—Unrecordable distal perfusion pressure or flat plethysmographic trace

B. Rutherford *et al.*[9] Ad hoc Committee on Reporting Standards, Society for Vascular Surgery/North American Chapter, International Society for Cardiovascular Surgery

		Capillary return	*Muscle weakness*	*Sensory loss*	*Dopplers*	
					Arterial	*Venous*
Viable	Not immediately threatened	Intact	None	None	Audible AP > 30 mmHg	Audible
Threatened	Salvageable	Slow	Partial	Mild	Inaudible	Audible
Irreversible	Tissue loss needs amputation	Absent (marbled)	Paralysis	Anaesthetic	Inaudible	Inaudible

AP = ankle pressure.

length of the occlusion and the presence of run off are often difficult to record accurately on emergency angiograms where the distal vessels are poorly visualized; however the severity of ischaemia can be assessed objectively using clinical examination and Doppler evaluation. Two definitions of acute critical ischaemia have been proposed[8,9] (Table 11.2). Following a prospective evaluation of these definitions in Nottingham, the following grading system was recommended in acute leg ischaemia.

Acute limb ischaemia (Nottingham 1990)[10]
Arrest of the circulation in a limb which previously had adequate perfusion at rest:

1. Acute critical ischaemia – no audible Doppler flow, flat plethysmographic trace, often a neuro-sensory deficit.
2. Acute sub-critical ischaemia – audible ankle blood flow, motor and sensory powers usually intact.

In a prospective study of 119 patients with acute leg ischaemia, outcome was compared in patients with acute critical ischaemia versus sub-critical ischaemia according to the definitions above. Limb salvage rates (37% vs. 78%, $P = 0.0001$) and mortality (43% vs. 5%, $P = 0.0001$), respectively, were significantly different between these groups[10]. This objective assessment using Doppler pressures has been shown to be strongly linked to limb outcome and is a useful method of grading risk. The presence of a neurological deficit on clinical examination is a sign that irreversible muscle necrosis is imminent and indicates that urgent treatment is required. Many patients have a slight degree of sensory loss at presentation and this does not imply such impending necrosis. It is an indication that prompt treatment is required but there is usually time for thrombolysis.

Information from randomized trials

There have been few well-constructed randomized trials in acute peripheral arterial ischaemia so they are worth analysing in some detail.

There are two trials which compare surgery and thrombolysis. The first by Graor *et al.* was not randomized but was a case-controlled study of thrombectomy versus initial thrombolysis for vascular graft occlusion[11]. Twenty-two patients received low-dose t-PA infusions and 38 matched patients were initially treated surgically. The results were 86% patency after lysis and 42% after surgery. However, 91% patients initially treated by thrombolysis required a secondary surgical procedure to revise and correct the underlying graft defect. Operation on a patent graft which has been reopened by lysis was more successful than primary surgical treatment and the authors concluded that the combination of thrombolysis and surgery is optimal.

Neilsson reported results of a randomized trial comparing thrombolysis using t-PA and initial surgery in 20 cases of native vessel arterial thrombosis[12]. Only six of 11 patients initially treated with thrombolysis had a good result compared with eight of nine treated surgically, though no statistical differences in outcome were found as all but one patient ultimately had limb salvage. Comparisons of surgery and thrombolysis are the most difficult of all investigations because such large numbers of patients are required to allow for the great variation in clinical details. Randomized trials have been commenced in the UK and the USA (The STILE study) but neither has yet reported results. Surgery and thrombolysis are not competing alternatives, but complementary. Surgery after initial thrombolysis is easier and probably safer than vice versa.

Detailed comparisons of thrombolytic agents have previously been discussed in Chapter 8. Most of the studies were not randomized and comparison of the costs of thrombolytic agents was often highlighted. A single small randomized trial emphasized superiority of t-PA over streptokinase[13]. Much anecdotal evidence is available for the superiority of t-PA over streptokinase, but large randomized trials have not been performed. The cost of the thrombolytic agent is such a small part of an admission for acute leg ischaemia that this is almost irrelevant. As yet major studies evaluating the cost effectiveness of the different thrombolytic agents have yet to be performed[14]. The fact that fibrin-specific drugs such as t-PA have failed to establish superiority and that there is still controversy is surprising[15] (Figure 11.2).

In conclusion randomized trials in acute leg ischaemia are extremely hard to organize and complete. Almost invariably they are too small to give significant information. It is important that the challenge is seized to undertake multi-centre studies and include formal cost-benefit analysis of thrombolysis. This has been achieved for femoro-distal reconstruction in critical limb ischaemia and a similar model could be used[16].

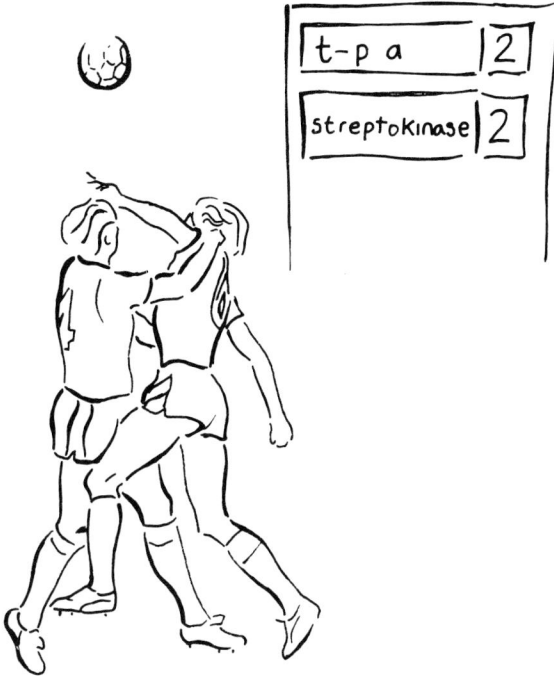

Figure 11.2 Peripheral thrombolysis: which agent is superior?

Future investigation

From the available information there is a good idea of high- and low-risk cases for thrombolytic therapy. Careful case selection is the most important predictor of outcome and it would be helpful to have additional objective methods of assessing the severity of ischaemia. Thrombus imaging and ageing techniques may provide information on its suitability for lysis. Thrombus imaging is in its infancy but monoclonal anti-platelet antibodies can be shown to accumulate at the site of recent thrombus and might be used to predict the 'lysability' of an occlusion[17]. Sophisticated ultrasonic techniques can also be used to investigate, and possibly age intra-lumenal thrombus[18]. New methods of assessing the severity of muscle ischaemia such as magnetic resonance spectrophotometry could be useful objective tests to determine the reversability of ischaemia. The main problem is that it is difficult to arrange these investigations out of hours when patients with acute leg ischaemia often present. Investigations may be particularly helpful in acute sub-critical ischaemia where more time is available.

The optimal thrombolytic agent can only be answered by randomized studies. The ideal method of administration – high dose or low dose – may be harder to determine because each method may be appropriate in different patients. For example if time is available and the patient is relatively high risk, a low-dose infusion over a day or two may be the safest method. Accelerated thrombolytic techniques may be indicated in acute critical ischaemia and possibly also for graft thrombosis, though formal studies will be required.

Modern management of acute leg ischaemia should include a more rigorous evaluation of the patient's medical condition. Early recognition of patients unlikely to benefit from intervention would be helpful[19]. In particular, cardiac function is a major predictor of outcome and this can easily be assessed by non-invasive measurement of cardiac output by Doppler methods. Early risk stratification is possible and Jivegard has evaluated an index which predicts death after embolectomy where patients at high risk have the following indicators: hypotension, cardiac failure, ischaemia involving the thigh, haemo-concentration and recent myocardial infarction[20].

Turning peripheral thrombolysis into a science

In order to perform multi-centre studies clinicians need to adopt a common approach and common aims. A Thrombolysis Study Group has been formed in the UK by interested vascular surgeons and radiologists with the following aims:

1. Collection of information on thrombolysis. It has been agreed to collect data from several centres in the UK and create a large database. With this information it is hoped to have a powerful tool with which to answer some of the key questions in thrombolysis. The group can discuss and disseminate any information discovered and audit each of their own results. It is hoped to be able to set standards in peripheral thrombolysis and publish guidelines and recommendations with authority. It is important that acceptable risks and hazards can be identified and quantified.
2. Standardize definitions. There is enormous variation in the methods used to describe results of thrombolytic treatments. Initially the group designed a database collection sheet using standardized definitions which is presently being used prospectively (Fig. 11.3). In particular defining results, outcome and complications has been difficult.
3. Perform randomized trials. It is important that this forum is used to determine which are the appropriate randomized studies to be performed and then to use a multi-centre approach. Until these are reported, sufficient information cannot be assembled to argue against an 'all surgery' approach to acute leg ischaemia[21].

Medico-legal aspects of thrombolysis trials

Thrombolytic agents do not have a product licence for use in peripheral thrombolysis, although this may be forthcoming. Clinicians who perform randomized trials into thrombolytic therapy can benefit from a common approach as documented by the Thrombolysis Study Group and benefit from the independence of that institution. Informed consent is difficult in patients with acute leg ischaemia who are often elderly and in pain, and who may be confused. An attempt should be made to try and explain the risks and hazards of the procedure, if not to the patient, then to a close relative. The haemorrhagic complications of thrombolysis are often emphasized in this discussion. It is worth remembering that similar risks are associated with major vascular reconstructions.

A contemporary approach

The following guidelines can be used to manage patients with acute leg ischaemia in hospitals equipped with on-call vascular radiology and a team approach to acute leg ischaemia. The thrombolytic options include standard low-dose infusions and accelerated infusion of thrombolytic agents which certainly expands the number of patients who can be treated.

When to operate

Patients with a brief history of ischaemia, an obvious embolic source and no prior history of claudication and an ilio-femoral occlusion fare very well from an embolectomy under local anaesthetic. If embolectomy is reserved for these cases, results will be good but the operation will seldom be performed. Patients with acute critical ischaemia including a neurological deficit need urgent treatment and in many cases the most appropriate method is by prompt surgical exploration. On-table angiography is easily performed if necessary and intra-operative thrombolysis is available as required. Intra-operative thrombolysis is useful in any situation where there is distal thrombus or embolus but is particularly indicated after failed embolectomy, for thrombosed popliteal aneurysms where it may become the procedure of choice and for 'trash foot'.[22] Angioscopic embolectomy may come to assume a greater role[23].

When to use thrombolysis

STANDARD LOW-DOSE INFUSION

This regimen is tried and tested in patients with acute sub-critical ischaemia and can expect to result in resolution of the occlusion in two-thirds of cases.

ACCELERATED INFUSION

This technique may be used as standard though it may be particularly indicated in patients with acute critical ischaemia and patients with graft thrombosis. The main problem is that it is labour intensive and requires a radiologist in a vascular radiology suite for several hours. This technique is still relatively untested but results and complications may worsen if there is any relaxation in case selection[24]. It is uncertain yet whether complications such as distal embolization, bleeding due to the higher dose or renal failure due to revascularization of severely ischaemic legs will be a problem[25]. Adjunctive methods such as clot aspiration and pulse spray lysis may find an expanding role as endovascular therapy increases and becomes more sophisticated[26].

THROMBOLYSIS RECORD FORM   PAGE 1

Please photocopy and send to database coordinator when completed

HOSPITAL (   )   TRIAL (   )

DETAILS

INITIALS (   )   HOSP. NO. (   )   D.O.B. (   )   SEX (   )

RISK FACTORS

SPECIFIC MEDICATIONS

ASPIRIN	B-BLOCKER	WARFARIN

ISCHAEMIC HEART DIS	DIABETES
P. VASC DISEASE	STROKE

PREVIOUS THROMBOLYSIS OR
ARTERIAL SURGERY   ASA

(   )   *GIVE DATE AND DETAILS*   (   )

DATE OF ADMISSION (   )

HISTORY OF EVENT
AND CLINICAL EXAM

| SITE | RL | LL | RA | LA | DURATION (   ) hours   FONTAINE | IIb | III | IV | ABPI (   )

INAUDIBLE (   )

CLINICAL CAUSE

THROMBUS	EMBOLUS	?
OTHER		*Specify*

SENSORY IMPAIRMENT

NONE	PARTIAL	COMPLETE

RADIOLOGY AND THROMBOLYSIS   INTRAOPERATIVE? (   )

TRANSFER FINDINGS
OF PRE AND POST
LYSIS TO
ARTERIAL MAPS.
For grafts, use
customised maps.

NATIVE VESSEL
GRAFT

IN SITU	REVERSED	PTFE	DACRON	COMPOSITE	

THROMBOLYSIS
START TIME
AND DATE   (   )

AGENT	STREPTOKINASE
	UROKINASE
	t-PA

CATHETER SIZE
SHEATH SIZE   (   )

OTHER DRUGS GIVEN,
INCLUDE DOSE
REGIMEN

*e.g. Heparin
or Praxilene*

TIME AND DATE
THROMBOLYSIS   (   )
STOPPED

TOTAL DOSE   (   )
GIVEN

INFUSION

DETAIL CHANGE IN INFUSION RATES

ROUTE | IV |— DOSE RATE (   ) mg/hr   INITIAL DOSE(S)

| IA |— METHOD

| INFUSION |
| BOLUS |
| PULSE SPRAY |

Then   FOR (   )
mg/hr   (   ) hr

Then   FOR (   )
mg/hr   (   ) hr

Then   FOR (   )
mg/hr   (   ) hr

Then   FOR (   )
mg/hr   (   ) hr

BOLUS SIZE, INTERVAL
AND INFUSION TIME
*e.g. 3 * 5mg over 15 mins*

(a)

THROMBOLYSIS RECORD FORM – OUTCOME DETAILS

Please photocopy and send to database coordinator when completed

TRIAL

INITIALS

HOSP. NO.

DATE OF THROMBOLYSIS

WERE THERE ANY COMPLICATIONS? IF YES COMPLETE SECTION
IF NO, GO TO INITIAL OUTCOME

PUNCTURE SITE

GI

RETROPERITONEAL

EMBOLIC

HAEMORHAGIC

CT confirmed

COMPLICATIONS

MAJOR BLEED (See definition over)	GROIN HAEMATOMA ALTERING MANAGEMENT	STROKE	EMBOLISATION
PERICATHETER THROMBOSIS	REPERFUSION INJURY/ RENAL FAILURE NEEDING Rx	ALLERGY/ANAPHYLAXIS	
DEATH SPECIFY: Describe relation if any to thrombolysis		DID THROMBOLYSIS HAVE TO BE STOPPED BECAUSE OF A COMPLICATION?	
OTHER		IF YES, AT WHAT TIME?	

RADIOLOGICAL OUTCOME

COMPLETE LYSIS	CLINICALLY USEFUL LYSIS	LYSIS BUT NO RUN-OFF/FLOW	NO LYSIS

ADJUNCTIVE MEASURES

POST LYSIS MEDICATION	HEPARIN- ASPIRIN	HEPARIN- WARFARIN	ASPIRIN	

SURGERY

RADIOLOGY

OTHER

NONE

SPECIFY

30 DAY OUTCOME

DID THE VESSEL RETHROMBOSIS?

YES

NO

DESCRIBE FURTHER PROCEDURES AFTER RETHROMBOSIS IN COMMENTS BOX

IF FURTHER LYSIS, COMPLETE NEW FORM

LIMB SURVIVAL

MAJOR AMPUTATION

DEATH

CAUSE

FONTAINE

ABPI

COMPLETE IF PERFORMED

SUMMARY/COMMENTS

(b)

ANGIOGRAPHIC APPEARANCE
Initial/End of thrombolysis/Time =
Delete and complete as required

Patient initials ⬭

Hosp. No. ⬭

Shade arterial map as follows:

☐ PATENT

▨ OCCLUDED

Identify the following with a mark to show its site:

⟨⟩ ANEURYSM

Max diam. = ☐

SFA diam. = ☐

Dist. Pop Diameter = ☐

)(STENOSIS

Percentage = ☐

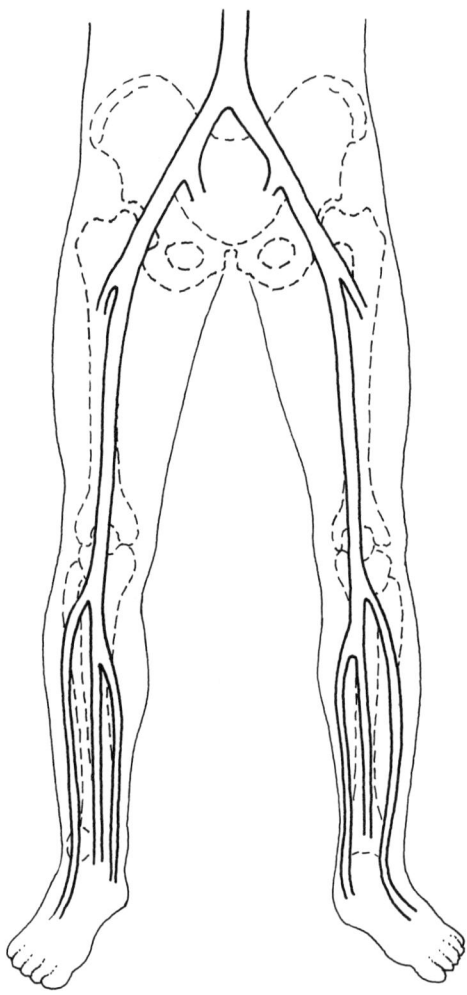

Complete one map before thrombolysis is started and one when completed. Photocopy and return to database coordinator.

(c)

Figure 11.3 (a)–(c) Thrombolysis record form (Thrombolysis Study Group)

Conclusion

Considering the first major investigations into peripheral thrombolysis began little more than a decade ago, tremendous advances in knowledge have been made. Intra-arterial thrombolysis has become widely accepted in most hospitals in the UK (and worldwide) as part of a multidisciplinary approach to acute leg ischaemia. That it has is a tribute to the pioneering enthusiasm of a few surgeons and radiologists who embraced the concept of thrombolysis and who undertook its evaluation. This work has had other benefits. It stimulated technical developments in other surgical and radiological fields and promoted a better understanding between vascular surgeons and radiologists. This book marks the end of the first phase of investigation into peripheral thrombolysis. The many open trials performed have often raised more questions than answers but have provided the framework with which to set an agenda for future studies. Like laparoscopic surgical techniques which have become widely established without careful evaluation because of clear clinical advantages, endovascular techniques such as thrombolysis and aspiration embolectomy require balanced evaluation. The challenge is there over the next few years to copy others such as the cardiologists with their large-scale coronary trials, to move forward constructively and collectively.

The importance of the challenge lies in the serious epidemiological problem which is looming. The number of elderly people is gradually increasing. Deaths from cardiovascular disease and diabetes have progressively fallen due to benefits of medical therapy. All these trends indicate there will be an increasing number of elderly patients with legs at risk from acute ischaemia. The morbidity of this condition is high and further evaluation of non-surgical techniques urgent.

There is no doubt that many legs have been saved by thrombolysis. Optimal management of acute leg ischaemia is by a combination of medical, endovascular and surgical treatment, combining clinical input from vascular surgeons and radiologists. A team approach to this and other vascular diseases will need to be developed over the coming years. The boundaries between disciplines such as surgery and radiology will become less distinct. This process may be uncomfortable but it is essential that turf battles are avoided.

The management of acute leg ischaemia will depend on local facilities and there are hospitals in the UK where this lags behind present ideals. In future, it may be appropriate that the majority of cases of acute leg ischaemia are initially treated by thrombolysis and clot aspiration, with surgery reserved for those in whom it fails. This will require a large expansion in the number of radiology and vascular surgery specialists. Justification for this expansion can only come from cost-benefit analysis of both surgical and non-surgical methods. Research initiatives which are presently being developed will need to provide data to justify the overwhelming clinical impression that thrombolysis is indeed a valuable treatment. The results of investigations performed over the next decade will determine the ultimate role of thrombolysis for acute leg ischaemia.

References

1. Buckenham TM, George CD, Chester JF, Taylor RS and Dormandy JA. Accelerated thrombolysis using pulsed intra-thrombus recombinant human tissue-type plasminogen activator. *Eur J Vasc Surg* 1992; **6**: 237–40
2. Walker WJ and Giddings AEB. A protocol for the safe treatment of acute lower limb ischaemia with intra-arterial streptokinase and surgery. *Br J Surg* 1988; **75**: 1189–92
3. Nachbur B. Treatment of acute ischaemia: every general surgeon's business? *Eur J Vasc Surg* 1988; **2**: 281–2
4. Walker WJ and Giddings AEB. Thrombolysis – a challenge for radiologists and surgeons. *Clin Radiol* 1990; **41**: 299–300
5. Earnshaw JJ and Shaw JFL. A survey of the use of thrombolysis for acute limb ischaemia in the UK and Ireland. *Br J Surg* 1990; **77**: 1041–2
6. Browse DJ, Barr H, Torrie EPH and Galland RB. Limitations to the widespread usage of low dose intra-arterial thrombolysis. *Eur J Vasc Surg* 1991; **5**: 445–9
7. Ricotta JJ, Green RM and DeWeese JA. Use and limitations of thrombolytic therapy in the treatment of peripheral arterial ischaemia: a multi-institutional questionnaire. *J Vasc Surg* 1987; **6**: 45–50
8. Bell PRF, Charlesworth D and DePalma RG et al. The definition of critical ischaemia of a limb. *Br J Surg* 1982; **69** (suppl): s2
9. Rutherford RB, Flanigan DP and Gupta SK et al. Suggested standards for reports dealing with lower extremity ischaemia. *J Vasc Surg* 1986; **4**: 80–94
10. Earnshaw JJ, Hopkinson BR and Makin GS. Acute critical ischaemia of the limb: a prospective evaluation. *Eur J Vasc Surg* 1990; **4**: 365–8
11. Graor RA, Risius B, Young JR et al. Thrombolysis of peripheral arterial bypass grafts: surgical thrombectomy compared with thrombolysis. *J Vasc Surg* 1988; **7**: 347–55
12. Nilsson L, Albrechtsson U and Jonung T et al. Surgical treatment versus thrombolysis in acute arterial occlusion: a randomized controlled study. *Eur J Vasc Surg* 1992; **6**: 189–93
13. Berridge DC, Gregson RHS, Hopkinson BR and Makin GS. Randomized trial of intra-arterial recombinant tissue plasminogen activator, intravenous recombinant tissue plasminogen activator and intra-arterial streptokinase in peripheral arterial thrombolysis. *Br J Surg* 1991; **78**: 988–95
14. Cronenwett JL, Dacey LJ, McDaniel MD, Walsh DB and Zwolak RM. Cost-effectiveness of intra-arterial thrombolytic therapy. *Br J Surg* 1988; **75**: 1265
15. Gaffney P. Tissue plasminogen activator for thrombolytic therapy: expectation versus reality. *J Roy Soc Med* 1992; **85**: 692–8
16. Cheshire NJW, Wolfe JHN, Noone MA, Davies L and Drummond M. The economics of femorocrural reconstruction for critical leg ischaemia with and without autologous vein. *J Vasc Surg* 1992; **15**: 167–75
17. Berridge DC, Perkins AC, Frier M et al. Detection and characterization of arterial thromboses using a platelet-specific monoclonal antibody. *Br J Surg* 1991; **78**: 1130–3
18. Parsons RE, Sigel B and Feleppa EJ et al. Age determination of experimental venous thrombi by ultrasonic tissue characterization. *J Vasc Surg* 1993; **17**: 470–8
19. Dreglid EB, Stangeland LB, Eide GE and Trippestad A. Patient survival and limb prognosis after arterial embolectomy. *Eur J Vasc Surg* 1987; **1**: 263–71
20. Jivegard L, Bergqvist D and Holm J et al. Preoperative assessment of the risk for cardiac death following thromboembolectomy for acute lower limb ischaemia. *Eur J Vasc Surg* 1992; **6**: 83–8
21. Allen DR, Smallwood J and Johnson CD. Intra-arterial thrombolysis should be the initial treatment of the acutely ischaemic lower limb. *Ann R Coll Surg Engl* 1992; **74**: 106–11
22. Earnshaw JJ and Beard JD. Intraoperative use of thrombolytic agents. *Br Med J* 1993; **307**: 638–9
23. White GH, White RA, Kopchok GE and Wilson SE. Angioscopic embolectomy: preliminary observations with a recent technique. *J Vasc Surg* 1988; **7**: 318–25
24. Braithwaite BD, Birch P, Davies C, Poskitt KR, Heather BP and Earnshaw JJ. Accelerated

high-dose bolus tissue plasminogen activator extends the role of peripheral thrombolysis but may increase risk. *Br J Surg* 1994; **81**: 619

25. Hartley R and Earnshaw JJ. Calcaneal necrosis secondary to distal embolization: a rare complication of peripheral intra-arterial thrombolysis. *Eur J Vasc Surg* (in press)

26. Wagner H-J and Starck EE. Acute embolic occlusions of the infrainguinal arteries: percutaneous aspiration embolectomy in 102 patients. *Radiology* 1992; **182**: 403–7

Index